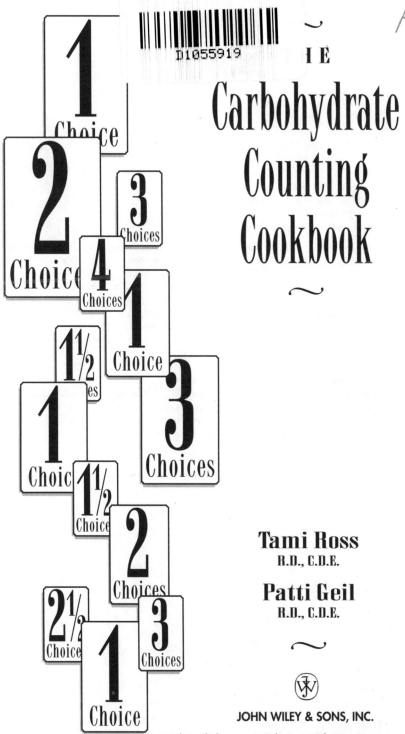

THE

Carbohydrate Counting Cookbook

~

Tami Ross
R.D., C.D.E.

Patti Geil
R.D., C.D.E.

~

JOHN WILEY & SONS, INC.

New York • Chichester • Weinheim • Brisbane • Singapore • Toronto

ISBN 0-471-34671-3

Printed in the United States of America

10 9 8 7 6 5 4 3

Contents

~

To Mike, Andrew, Mom, Dad, and Gran—my number one taste testers—who throughout the creation of this book consumed more grams of carbohydrate than I can count! Thanks for your support and input!   —T.A.R.

To Jack, Kristen, and Rachel, who I always count on!   —P.B.G.

To Jeff Braun—many thanks for your enthusiasm, guidance, and support along the way. We've managed to survive disasters, both natural and in the kitchen, during the writing of this book. Your personal concern and attention to detail are much appreciated!

Counting Carbohydrates

The New Approach to Eating

Beverly has had Type 1 diabetes for 13 years. She is a busy, young, married professional. Beverly and her husband want to start a family in the near future. She feels she has been fairly successful with her diabetes management. Beverly takes two shots of insulin a day, follows a no-concentrated-sweets diet, and checks her blood sugar every morning. However, her life has become more hectic and she finds it difficult to eat on time. As a result, she frequently experiences low-blood-sugar reactions, which she treats by eating a small bag of M&M's. Her blood sugar then rises and often stays high. Beverly is tired of riding the blood sugar roller coaster.

Bill is a 52-year-old accountant who was recently diagnosed with Type 2 diabetes. He takes an oral diabetes medication, walks for exercise almost every day, and tries to eat less sugar and fat now that he has diabetes. Bill checks his blood-sugar level in the morning and before supper. He notices that his afternoon blood-sugar levels are higher during the week and wonders if it's due to the fast food lunch he eats on workdays.

Two different people, two different types of diabetes, two different life-styles. Can a single approach to eating work for both of them?

Improving Your Blood Sugar Control

Carbohydrate counting may be just the answer for both Beverly and Bill. And it may be what you need to improve your blood-sugar control, while adding flexibility to your food choices. Counting the grams of carbohydrate in your food is a very precise method of meal planning, which helps keep your blood-sugar levels in control.

Carbohydrate-containing foods, such as grains, vegetables, fruit, and milk, have the most immediate impact on blood sugar. Ninety percent of the digestible starches and sugars we eat appear in the blood as glucose (blood sugar) within two hours after eating. Eating small amounts of carbohydrate will raise blood sugar; eating larger amounts of carbohydrate will raise blood sugar even more.

The 1994 Nutrition Recommendations for People With Diabetes opens new doors by noting that it is more important to eat a consistent amount of carbohydrate at meals and snacks rather than focus on the type of carbohydrate eaten. Research shows that sugar does not raise blood sugar any more than the same amount of starch. This means that you can eat foods containing sugar as long as you count them toward the total carbohydrate allotment for that meal or snack. In fact, you'll find that several of the recipes in this cookbook contain small amounts of sugar, formerly considered off limits for people with diabetes. Testing your blood sugar 1 1/2 to 2 hours after you eat will help you target the ideal amount of carbohydrate to eat. Eating a consistent amount of carbohydrate from day to day, when combined with exercise and diabetes medication if necessary, will improve your blood-sugar control.

Because a carbohydrate is a carbohydrate is a carbohydrate, if you use the carbohydrate-counting approach you can eat foods from garlic bread to chocolate chip cookies in moderate amounts, as long as you account for the number of grams of carbohydrate. As an added benefit, your diabetes medication will no longer dictate when and what you should eat. Instead, your food choices will determine your medication dosage and timing.

Why This Cookbook?

Carbohydrate counting is easy to learn and use in planning your meals and snacks. Normally, it involves taking the time to accurately determine food portion sizes, calculating the amount of carbohydrate in your foods, and testing your blood sugar after you eat. *The Carbohydrate Counting Cookbook*, however, eliminates much of the effort.

Regularly testing your blood sugar is still important. But with each of these family-tested recipes, there will be no guesswork regarding portion sizes or carbohydrate amounts. *The Carbohydrate Counting Cookbook* is designed to make it easy for you to include new recipes in your meal plan. The number of carbohydrate choices and grams of carbohydrate contained in a serving are highlighted in the nutrition information provided with each recipe.

Sample menus (page 193) based on an 1800 calorie diet show you can see ways to combine the recipes in *The Carbohydrate Counting Cookbook* to keep your carbohydrate intake consistent from day to day.

Recipe listings (page 195) are arranged so recipes with an equal number of carbohydrate choices are grouped together. If you want to plan a meal of six carbohydrate choices, use Appendix 2 to help you mix and match.

While the following pages offer an introduction to carbohydrate counting, educational sessions with a registered dietitian and your health care team will provide you with valuable information about the more detailed aspects of carbohydrate counting. Whether you are a beginner or experienced carbohydrate counter, *The Carbohydrate Counting Cookbook* is meant to inspire you with delicious recipes to improve your diabetes control.

Why Count Carbohydrates?

Research from the Diabetes Control and Complications Trial proves that better blood-sugar control reduces the risk of complications from diabetes, including nerve damage, damage to the eyes, and kidney disease. And healthy eating is a major part of good blood-sugar control. You have many nutrition options, ranging from simple guidelines based on the food pyramid to the exchange system to carbohydrate counting.

If you have Type 1 diabetes and use the carbohydrate counting approach, you will be able to determine how much insulin you require when you eat a certain amount of carbohydrate. You will come to appreciate the increased flexibility in the timing of your meals and snacks. People with Type 2 diabetes will benefit from the improved blood-sugar control that comes from consistent carbohydrate intake.

The importance of counting carbohydrate has been apparent for some time. In 1935, the famed diabetes physician Elliott P. Joslin said, "In teaching patients their diet, I lay emphasis first on carbohydrate values, and teach to a few only the values for protein and fat."

The goal of carbohydrate counting is to improve your blood-sugar control by matching the amount of carbohydrate you eat to the amount of insulin available. It enables people with diabetes to learn the quantity of carbohydrate their body can use without raising blood-sugar levels too much.

The Recipes

The recipes in *The Carbohydrate Counting Cookbook* are meant to be enjoyed by everyone in your family—not just the person with diabetes! The 1994 Nutrition Recommendations for People with Diabetes stress that eating right with diabetes involves following the same nutritional guidelines for all healthy Americans:

- Eat a variety of foods.
- Balance the food you eat with physical activity—maintain or improve your weight.
- Choose a diet with plenty of grain products, vegetables, and fruit.
- Choose a diet low in fat, saturated fat, and cholesterol.
- Choose a diet moderate in sugars.
- Choose a diet moderate in salt and sodium.
- If you drink alcoholic beverages, do so in moderation.

We've chosen our recipes to meet these guidelines as part of an overall well-balanced diet. The recipes have passed the taste and time-crunch tests of our busy families and friends, who, like you, appreciate having a fast, yet healthy, meal on the table.

When selecting your favorites, note the nutrition information and special markings:

Recipes that are high in sodium (more than 400 mg per serving) are marked with an **S**. Use these recipes occasionally, particularly if you are following a sodium-restricted meal plan.

Recipes that are high in fiber (more than 5 grams per serving.) are marked with an **F**. Remember to take the fiber content of a meal into consideration when calculating your carbohydrate intake, as noted on page 14.

How Does Carbohydrate Counting Work?

If you decide carbohydrate counting is for you, there are two approaches to consider. For either approach, a few sessions with a registered dietitian will provide you with valuable information and support as you learn this new method of meal planning.

The first basic approach involves setting a target carbohydrate goal for each meal and snack. This allows flexibility in food choices while providing consistent carbohydrate intake and is a good approach for people with Type 2 diabetes. For example, after discussing his typical eating pattern with a registered dietitian, Bill set a target of 40 grams of carbohydrate at breakfast, 40 grams of carbohydrate at lunch, 60 grams of carbohydrate at supper and 30 grams of carbohydrate for his evening snack. In practice, Bill finds that it doesn't seem to matter whether the 40 grams of carbohydrate at breakfast comes from fruit, bread, or milk. His blood sugars remain in control when he keeps the total amount of carbohydrate at breakfast consistent from day to day.

Another approach to carbohydrate counting, appropriate for people with Type 1 diabetes, involves calculating your own personal carbohydrate-to-insulin ratio. This is the measurement of the amount of carbohydrate you metabolize with one unit of insulin. When Beverly began carbohydrate counting, her physician recommended she take an injection of a long-acting insulin (such as Ultralente) every morning as a basal dose to cover her nonfood insulin needs. With the help of careful blood-sugar testing and record keeping, Beverly finds that her diabetes control is best when she also injects one unit of fast-acting insulin for every 15 grams of carbohydrate in her meal. For example, if her lunch contains 60 grams of carbohydrate, she takes 4 units of regular insulin one-half hour before she eats. If Beverly wants to eat an additional serving of mashed potatoes, she keeps in mind that 1/2 cup of mashed potatoes has approximately 15 grams of carbohydrate. Therefore, she knows she will require one extra unit of regular insulin at that meal. Carbohydrate counting allows Beverly more flexibility in her food choices. In addition, if her schedule changes and her meal is delayed, she can adjust the timing of her insulin injection as well.

Carbohydrate counting is not an invitation to a nutrition free-for-all. While you can now include small amounts of sweets in your meal plan, making the mistake of ignoring good nutrition principles can lead to consequences such as weight gain and high blood-fat levels. Healthy food choices should be the main consideration, no matter which meal planning approach is used. Also, keep in mind that your tolerance for carbohydrate may change over time, so your carbohydrate goal and carbohydrate-to-insulin ratio are not set in stone. Factors such as exercise, medications, pregnancy, weight gain, and physical activity can alter your carbohydrate requirements.

Getting Started: Easy as 1, 2, 3

1.Which Foods Contain Carbohydrate? Carbohydrate is found in starches and sugars. Foods that contain carbohydrate include breads, crackers, and cereals; pasta, rice, and grains; vegetables; milk and yogurt; fruit and juice; and table sugar, honey, syrup, and molasses, as well as foods sweetened with them.

Other foods, such as cake, ice cream, candy, snack foods, pizza, casseroles, and soups contain a combination of carbohydrate, protein, and fat.

Some foods, such as meat, fish, eggs, oils, cheese, bacon, butter, and margarine contain fat and/or protein, but have no carbohydrate.

Foods that don't have carbohydrate do not need to be accounted for in the carbohydrate counting approach because they don't raise blood sugar levels as much as carbohydrate foods do. Fat and protein still play a key role by delaying carbohydrate digestion and metabolism. The main focus of your meal plan should be healthy eating. Ignoring protein and fat can lead to poor nutrition, weight gain, and increased risk of heart disease and cancer.

Quick Quiz: Carbohydrate Hide and Seek

Fourteen of the 20 foods listed below contain carbohydrate. Can you find them?

Skim milk	Fruit cocktail
Kidney beans	Bacon
Whole wheat bagel	Raisins
Carrot sticks	Peanut butter
Hard boiled egg	Glazed doughnut
Pasta salad	Canola oil
Pepperoni pizza	Oatmeal
Popcorn	Light beer
Cheddar cheese	Sour cream
Mayonnaise	Low fat yogurt

The correct answers can be found in the answer key on page 15.

---

2. Tools of the Trade Carbohydrate in foods is measured in grams, but it's not necessary to be a metric expert to try carbohydrate counting. Although a gram is a measure of weight, it may be more helpful to think of grams of carbohydrate as a measure of the blood-sugar-raising potential of the food. You cannot weigh a food and know the grams of carbohydrate it contains by weight alone. You must take the next step of using a reference book to assist you in calculating the amount of carbohydrate in the food.

Putting carbohydrate counting to work requires having the right tools and resources. Because carbohydrate counting is based on portion sizes, first on the list are food scales, measuring cups, and measuring spoons. Even small measurements such as ounces and tablespoons make a difference.

Measuring Up

Note the difference in the amount of carbohydrate when you measure a food exactly, versus using common kitchen dishes, cups, and glasses to track portion sizes.

8 ounces of skim milk=12 grams of carbohydrate
Glass of skim milk=18 grams of carbohydrate

1 ounce of cornflakes=24 grams of carbohydrate
Bowl of cornflakes=48 grams of carbohydrate

1 cup of pasta=40 grams of carbohydrate
Plate of pasta=120 grams of carbohydrate

1 cup of green salad=5 grams of carbohydrate
Bowl of green salad=10 grams of carbohydrate

1 ounce (1/2) bagel=15 grams of carbohydrate
Bakery bagel=45 grams of carbohydrate

In addition to knowing exact portion sizes, knowing the amount of carbohydrate in a food is also crucial. The following list of resources will help you determine the carbohydrate content of the foods you eat:

The Diabetes Carbohydrate and Fat Gram Guide, Lea Ann Holzmeister, R.D., C.D.E., American Diabetes Association, 1997

Fast Food Facts, Fifth Edition, Marion Franz, M.S., R.D., C.D.E., International Diabetes Center, Inc., 1997

Food Values of Portions Commonly Used, Jean Pennington, J.B. Lippincott Company, 1997

Nutrition in the Fast Lane, Franklin Publishing, 1996

Carbohydrate Counting: Getting Started, Moving On, Using Carbohydrate/Insulin Ratios; and *Exchange Lists for Meal Planning,* American Diabetes Association, American Dietetic Association, 1995

Carbohydrate Gram Counter, Corrine Netzer, Dell Publishing, 1994

The Complete Book of Food Counts, Corrine Netzer, Dell Publishing/Bantam, 1994

Food labels also provide key information. As you read the food label below, look for these three things:

Nutrition Facts

Serving Size 1 cup (228g)
Servings Per Container 2

Amount Per Serving

Calories 260   Calories from Fat 120

	% Daily Value*
Total Fat 13g	20%
Saturated Fat 5g	25%
Cholesterol 30mg	10%
Sodium 660mg	28%
Total Carbohydrate 31g	10%
Dietary Fiber 0g	0%
Sugars 5g	
Protein 13g	•

Vitamin A 4%	•	Vitamin C 2%	
Calcium 15%	•	Iron 4%	

* Percent Daily Values are based on a 2,000 calorie diet. Your daily values may be higher or lower depending on your calorie needs:

		Calories:	2,000	2,500
Total Fat	Less than		65g	80g
Sat Fat	Less than		20g	25g
Cholesterol	Less than		300mg	300mg
Sodium	Less than		2,400mg	2,400mg
Total Carbohydrate			300g	375g
Dietary Fiber			25g	30g

Calories per gram:
Fat 9   •   Carbohydrate 4   •   Protein 4

The "Total Carbohydrate" section contains the information most relevant to carbohydrate counting—the total grams of carbohydrate per serving. There are 31 grams of total carbohydrate per serving in this example.

Pay attention to the serving size listed at the top of the label. The total carbohydrate information may be based on a serving size that is somewhat different than what you'd typically eat. If you ate 2 cups of the food on the sample label, you'd actually be consuming 62 grams of carbohydrate, rather than 31 grams.

Note the amount of fiber listed on the label. As explained on page 14, the amount of fiber in a serving of food may change the amount of carbohydrate available to be metabolized.

Carbohydrate Grams vs. Carbohydrate Choices: Which is Best for You?

Carbohydrate counting may be done in two ways: by calculating the exact number of grams of carbohydrate (CHO) in a food, meal, or snack, or by using the "carbohydrate choice" method. You can calculate the exact number of grams of carbohydrate you eat in a day by keeping detailed records of each food and its carbohydrate content. In the carbohydrate choice method, you keep track of the number of carbohydrate choices you eat each day. Fifteen grams of carbohydrate equals one carbohydrate choice. For example, 1 1/2 cups of pasta has 45 grams of carbohydrate; it counts as three carbohydrate choices. A small orange has 15 grams of carbohydrate, so it is equal to one carbohydrate choice. The sample meal below illustrates both methods of carbohydrate counting:

Food	Portion Size	Grams CHO	Number of CHO Choices
Fish fillet	3 ounces	0	0
Fresh corn	1/2 cup	15	1
Baked potato	1 small	15	1
Dinner roll	1 small	15	1
Fresh fruit salad	1 cup	15	1
Sorbet	1/2 cup	30	2
TOTAL		**90 grams**	**6 CHO Choices**

Both methods work well, but the carbohydrate gram method offers more precision, particularly if you are interested in calculating your carbohydrate-to-insulin ratio.

3. Count 'Em Up, Write It Down Once you select a method and have the right resources on hand, it's time to begin. Start by writing down your usual food intake, taking care to note exact portion sizes. Here's what a typical day's food record for Bill looks like:

Food	Portion Size	Grams of Carbohydrate
Scrambled egg	1 egg	<1
Bacon	3 slices	0
Toast	2 slices	26
Margarine	2 teaspoons	0
Coffee	1 cup	0
Double cheeseburger	1	31
French fries	Medium order	49
Diet soft drink	12 ounces	0
Grilled chicken breast	6 ounces	0
Rice pilaf	1/2 cup	30
Garden salad	1 small	5
Italian salad dressing	2 tablespoons	6
Watermelon	1 cup	12
Sugar-free iced tea	12 ounces	0
	TOTAL	**160 grams**

This amount of work may seem overwhelming at first, but good diabetes control is worth it. When you start out, you will have to spend a fair amount of time weighing and measuring foods, as well as calculating your actual intake. Begin keeping your own custom made list of favorite foods with carbohydrate content noted; this will save you the time of recalculating the carbohydrate content each time you enjoy a familiar recipe or food.

Keeping good records will help you achieve good blood-sugar control. Track the amount of carbohydrate you eat, the amount of medication you take and your blood-sugar results. With the help of your health care team, you can make the necessary adjustments for excellent blood-sugar control. For example, when Bill reviewed his food records, he realized that his fast food lunch of 80 grams of carbohydrate during the week was quite different from the 40 grams of carbohydrate in the smaller lunch of soup and salad that he ate on the weekends. Using the information from his food record enabled Bill to make adjustments and eat a consistent amount of carbohydrate from day to day. Consistency in carbohydrate intake leads to better blood-sugar control. To assist you in tracking your progress, there is a sample record-keeping form on page 16 that can be copied for your use. (Enlarge your copies to 200% for easier reading.)

Special Situations

No Free Lunch Beverly began using the carbohydrate-counting approach with great success. She learned to calculate the amount of insulin she took before meals based on the amount of carbohydrate she planned to eat. Beverly also learned some surprising things along the way. She had always included fat-free foods in her meal plan, assuming that they were also low in calories and carbohydrate. After reading several food labels, she realized that fat-free does not necessarily mean calorie-free or carbohydrate-free. In fact, some of her favorite fat-free foods were quite high in carbohydrate and calories:

Food	Carbohydrate	Calories
Fat-free ranch salad dressing (2 Tbsp.)	11 grams	50
Fat-free cream cheese (2 Tbsp.)	1 gram	25
Fat-free fig cookies (2)	22 grams	100
Fat-free vanilla ice cream (1/2 cup)	20 grams	90

Another eye-opener was the amount of carbohydrate in foods traditionally considered "free foods." When Beverly carefully measured the amount of lettuce, tomatoes, carrots, peppers, celery, and croutons in her dinner salad, she realized that she should be taking an additional unit of insulin to cover the 15 grams of carbohydrate in a food she had considered "free." This is another case in which careful carbohydrate counting can lead to better control.

Figure in Fiber Because fiber is a carbohydrate that is not digested or absorbed in the same way as sugar and starches, it does not turn into blood sugar. Therefore, a high fiber meal won't raise blood sugar as much as a lower fiber meal, even if both meals have the same amount of carbohydrate. Diabetes nutrition experts suggest the following rule of thumb: if there are 5 or more grams of fiber in a serving, subtract them from the total grams of carbohydrate to determine how much carbohydrate to count. For example, "Spicy Black Bean and Rice Soup" on page 130 has 11 grams of fiber per serving. You should subtract 11 grams from the grams of carbohydrate at that meal to find the amount of carbohydrate to count. In this cookbook, all recipes with 5 or more grams of fiber per serving are marked to remind you to figure in fiber.

Dinner at the Carbohydrate Counting Cafe Eating in restaurants is an American way of life. Chances are you eat at least three or four meals a week away from home. When you first learn about carbohydrate counting, it may seem hard to imagine calculating grams of carbohydrate in a restaurant setting. However, with a little preparation, carbohydrate counting can be taken on the road.

- **Practice at home.** Once you are able to estimate portion sizes accurately at home, you will know at a glance the amount of carbohydrate in your restaurant meal.

- **Scout out the menu ahead of time.** If possible, order a take out of your favorite restaurant foods so you can bring them home to weigh and measure. You'll know the carbohydrate content of the meal before you order next time.

- **If you live life in the fast-food lane, carbohydrate counting can work for you.** Nutrition information is yours for the asking from most fast-food restaurant chains. Here's a sampling of typical fast-food meals and their carbohydrate content:

Food	Portion Size	Grams of Carbohydrate
Sausage/egg biscuit	1	33
Hash browns	1 order	14
Coffee	12 ounces	0
TOTAL		**47 grams**
Pepperoni pizza	2 slices	45
Bread stick	1	20
Garden salad	1 serving	5
with reduced-calorie red		
French salad dressing	1 packet	23
Diet soft drink	12 ounces	0
TOTAL		**93 grams**
Fried chicken	1 breast	12
	1 drumstick	4
Cole slaw	1 order	13
Buttermilk biscuit	1	20
Sugar-free iced tea	12 ounces	0
TOTAL		**49 grams**

If you eat in fast-food restaurants often, don't focus on carbohydrate content alone and ignore the protein and fat content of your meals. The amount of fat found in fast food is not good for your overall health. Eating high-fat foods can also delay the absorption of the carbohydrate in your meal, which leads to unusual blood-sugar test results.

Answer Key

Quick Quiz: Carbohydrate Hide and Seek (page 8)

The 14 foods that contain carbohydrate are:

> Skim milk, kidney beans, whole wheat bagel, carrot sticks, pasta salad, pepperoni pizza, popcorn, fruit cocktail, raisins, peanut butter, glazed doughnut, oatmeal, light beer, and low fat yogurt

FOOD AND BEVERAGE RECORD

Day/Date: _____

Food and Amount	Grams CHO & #CHO Choices	Blood Sugar Level (Time)	Diabetes Medication (Time and Amount)	Comments (Physical Activity, Illness)
Breakfast Time: ____	Total: ____			
Snack Time: ____	Total: ____			
Lunch Time: ____	Total: ____			
Snack Time: ____	Total: ____			
Snack Time: ____	Total: ____			
Dinner Time: ____	Total: ____			
Snack Time: ____	Total: ____			

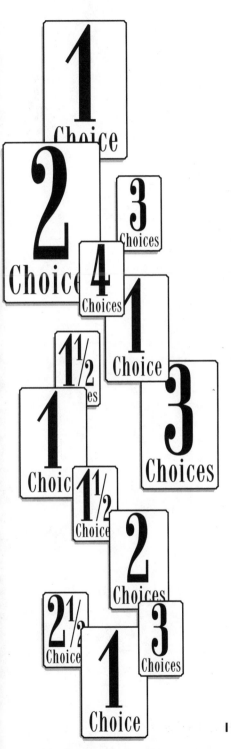

Beverages

Frosty Orange Frappé

This refreshing icy beverage is reminiscent of the Orange Julius.

6 ounces unsweetened frozen orange juice
   concentrate
1/2 cup skim milk
1 cup cold water
1 teaspoon vanilla extract
6 packets aspartame sweetener
18 ice cubes

Place first 5 ingredients in electric blender, cover, and combine
using frappé setting. Add ice cubes and frappé until icy smooth.
Serve immediately.

Makes 8 (4 fluid ounce) servings
Preparation time: 5 minutes

Nutrient Information (per serving):

Servings per recipe 8

Serving size 4 fluid ounces

Carbohydrate choices 1

Calories 44

Carbohydrate 10 grams

Protein 1 gram

Fat <1 gram

Saturated Fat <1 gram

Cholesterol <1 gram

Sodium 9 milligrams

Dietary Fiber <1 gram

% calories from:
   Protein 9%
   Carbohydrate 91%
   Fat 0

Food Exchanges: 1/2 skim milk

Icy Cinnamon Café

0 Choices

Iced coffee made its debut more than 120 years ago. Enjoy the hint of cinnamon in our version of this refreshing after-dinner treat! Recipe can easily be doubled.

- 1 cup cold coffee
- 2 packets saccharin sweetener (or 3 packets aspartame sweetener)
- 1/4 teaspoon ground cinnamon
- 4 cups crushed ice
- 4 teaspoons light whipped topping

Place coffee, sweetener, cinnamon, and ice in blender and blend until slushy. Pour into 4 glasses and top each with 1 teaspoon light whipped topping.

Note: While the percentage of fat calories appears high at 53%, note that there is only 1 gram of fat in this 17 calorie beverage.

Makes 4 (1 cup) servings
Preparation time: 5 minutes

Nutrient Information (per serving):

Servings per recipe 4	Cholesterol <1 milligram
Serving size 1 cup	Sodium 5 milligrams
Carbohydrate choices 0	Dietary Fiber 0
Calories 17	% calories from:
Carbohydrate 2 grams	Protein 0
Protein <1 gram	Carbohydrate 47%
Fat 1 gram	Fat 53%
Saturated Fat <1 gram	

Food Exchanges: Free

Lemon Mint Tea-ser

Serve over crushed ice or sugar-free lemonade "ice cubes."
Try making with decaf tea for a caffeine-free beverage.

3 cups water

6 regular-size tea bags

1/2 cup loosely packed chopped fresh mint leaves

2 packets sugar-free lemonade mix (enough to make 2 quarts lemonade)

8 cups cold water

Bring the 3 cups water to boil in a large saucepan. Remove from heat and add tea bags and mint. Steep for 15 minutes. Remove tea bags. Pour tea/mint through a sieve into a 2-quart pitcher; discard mint. Stir in lemonade mix and cold water. Refrigerate until chilled, about 1 hour.

Makes 11 (1 cup) servings
Preparation time: 5 minutes
Standing time: 15 minutes
Chilling time: 1 hour

Nutrient Information (per serving):

Servings per recipe 11	Cholesterol 0
Serving size 1 cup	Sodium 2 milligrams
Carbohydrate choices 0	Dietary Fiber 0
Calories 4	% calories from:
Carbohydrate 1 gram	Protein 0
Protein <1 gram	Carbohydrate 100%
Fat <1 gram	Fat 0
Saturated Fat <1 gram	

Food Exchanges: Free

Cranberry Sparkler

A beautiful punch to serve during the holidays or on any festive occasion. Float frozen cranberries in the punch to add a simple icy garnish.

- 2 quarts light cranberry juice
- 2-liter bottle diet ginger ale
- 1-liter bottle club soda

Combine in a large punch bowl and serve at once.

Makes 20 (1 cup) servings
Preparation time: 5 minutes

Nutrient Information (per serving):

Servings per recipe 20
Serving size 1 cup
Carbohydrate choices 0
Calories 16
Carbohydrate 4 grams
Protein 0
Fat 0
Saturated Fat 0

Cholesterol 0
Sodium 41 milligrams
Dietary Fiber 0
% calories from:
  Protein 0
  Carbohydrate 100%
  Fat 0

Food Exchanges: Free

Tomato Basil Warm-Up

½ Choice

S

Basil's rich, mildly pepper-like flavor complements the tangy tomato juice in this spicy beverage. Garnish each mug with a small celery stalk.

- 32-ounces canned tomato juice
- 16 ounces reduced-sodium, fat-free beef bouillon
- 1 tablespoon fresh-squeezed lemon juice
- 1/2 teaspoon dried basil

Combine all ingredients in a 2-quart pan and place over medium heat. Cook for 20 minutes, stirring periodically. Serve warm.

Note: Use reduced-sodium tomato juice to decrease the sodium content of this beverage.

Makes 6 (1 cup) servings
Preparation time: 5 minutes
Cooking time: 20 minutes

Nutrient Information (per serving):

Servings per recipe 6
Serving size 1 cup
Carbohydrate choices 1/2
Calories 41
Carbohydrate 8 grams
Protein 1 gram
Fat <1 gram
Saturated Fat <1 gram

Cholesterol 0
Sodium 574 milligrams
Dietary Fiber 1 gram
% calories from:
  Protein 10%
  Carbohydrate 78%
  Fat 12%

Food Exchanges: 2 vegetable

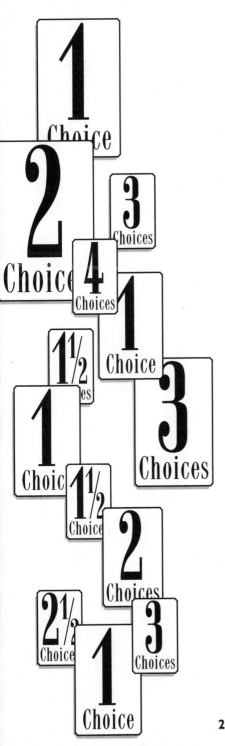

Appetizers

25

Buffalo Chicken Bites

*Celery sticks and reduced-fat ranch or blue cheese dressing
are a nice accompaniment to this fiery appetizer! To save time
during those precious last minutes before your party, combine
chicken chunks and sauce in the baking dish earlier in the day
and refrigerate. At party time you can quickly pop it into the
oven! Leftovers can be tossed with crispy, fresh lettuce for a
quick and filling salad.*

1 pound cooked chicken breasts, diced into bite-size chunks

Cooking spray

Sauce:

1/2 cup Red-Hot sauce

3 tablespoons melted reduced-calorie margarine

2 teaspoons chopped dried parsley

1/4 teaspoon garlic powder

Preheat oven to 350°. Place chicken bites in a baking dish coated
with cooking spray. In a bowl, combine sauce ingredients. Pour
sauce evenly over chicken and bake for 20 minutes. Put a toothpick in each piece of chicken and place on serving tray.

Makes 6 (7 piece) servings
Preparation time: 5 minutes
Baking time: 20 minutes

Nutrient Information (per serving):

Servings per recipe 6	Cholesterol 64 milligrams
Serving size 7 pieces chicken	Sodium 209 milligrams
Carbohydrate choices 0	Dietary Fiber <1 gram
Calories 154	% calories from:
Carbohydrate 1 gram	Protein 62 %
Protein 24 grams	Carbohydrate 3 %
Fat 6 grams	Fat 35 %
Saturated Fat 1 gram	

Food Exchanges: 3 lean meat

Cheesy Ham and Mushroom Quiche Bites

½
Choice

This richly flavored appetizer rendition of quiche freezes well. Warm up leftovers for breakfast.

1 1/2 cups liquid egg substitute
1 cup skim milk
1 cup biscuit baking mix
4 ounces finely shredded reduced-fat cheddar cheese
4 ounces finely shredded fat-free cheddar cheese
7-ounce can sliced mushrooms, drained
1 cup finely diced lean ham
1 small onion, finely diced
Cooking spray

Preheat oven to 400°. In a large bowl, whisk together egg substitute and milk. Stir in baking mix and cheeses, followed by mushrooms, ham, and onion. Spoon batter into 24 muffin cups coated with cooking spray. Bake for 20 minutes, or until toothpick inserted in muffin comes out clean. Turn out of pans promptly (may have to loosen edge of muffins with knife). Serve warm.

Makes 24 (1 muffin) servings
Preparation time: 15 minutes
Baking time: 20 minutes

Nutrient Information (per serving):

Servings per recipe 24	Cholesterol 5 milligrams
Serving size 1 muffin	Sodium 220 milligrams
Carbohydrate choices 1/2	Dietary Fiber 1 gram
Calories 62	% calories from:
Carbohydrate 5 grams	Protein 39%
Protein 6 grams	Carbohydrate 32%
Fat 2 grams	Fat 29%
Saturated Fat 1 gram	

Food Exchanges: 1 vegetable, 1 very lean meat

Tasty Tortilla Roll-Ups

Tortillas are the bread of Mexican cooking. Originally all tortillas were made from corn, but when the Spanish brought wheat to the New World, flour tortillas were created. Cowboys used to dine on stuffed tortillas around the crackling camp fire, but your party guests can sample these tortilla roll-ups alongside your cozy fire!

8-ounce package fat-free cream cheese

1/2 cup mild taco sauce

4-ounce can chopped green chilies, drained

5 green onions, finely chopped

10 (9-inch) fat-free flour tortillas

1 cup finely shredded reduced-fat cheddar cheese

Place cream cheese in a mixing bowl and whip with an electric mixer until light and fluffy. Blend in taco sauce, chilies, and onions. Spread cream cheese mixture on each of the flour tortillas. Sprinkle each with cheese. Roll up each tortilla, wrap with plastic wrap, place in airtight container, and refrigerate overnight to allow flavors to blend.

Before serving, unwrap tortilla, and slice each roll-up into 5 servings. Accompany with salsa for dipping.

Makes 25 (2 slice) servings
Preparation time: 20 minutes
Chilling time: 8 hours

Nutrient Information (per serving):

Servings per recipe 25

Serving size 2 slices

Carbohydrate choices 1/2

Calories 57

Carbohydrate 8 grams

Protein 4 grams

Fat 1 gram

Saturated Fat <1 gram

Cholesterol 3 milligrams

Sodium 255 milligrams

Dietary Fiber 2 grams

% calories from:

Protein 28%

Carbohydrate 56%

Fat 16%

Food Exchanges: 2 vegetable

Asparagus in Tangy Dijon Vinaigrette

Take care not to overcook the asparagus. This makes a pleasurable salad or side dish with a juicy grilled steak or a succulent pork roast!

Dijon Vinaigrette:

1 1/2 tablespoons red wine vinegar

4 tablespoons olive oil

1 1/2 teaspoons Dijon mustard

2 tablespoons fat-free sour cream

1/4 teaspoon salt

1/8 teaspoon coarse ground black pepper

2 pounds fresh asparagus, tough ends removed

Place vinaigrette ingredients in a blender, and blend until smooth. Set aside.

Place asparagus in a steamer pan over 2 inches boiling water. Cover and steam asparagus for 4 minutes, or until bright green and crisp-tender (may need to steam asparagus in two or three separate batches if steamer pan is small). Transfer asparagus from steamer to colander and place under cold running water to stop cooking process. Put steamed asparagus in a shallow serving dish and drizzle with the Dijon vinaigrette. Spread evenly over asparagus with the back of a spoon. Cover tightly with plastic wrap and refrigerate overnight, or for 8 hours, to allow flavors to blend.

Makes 6 (approximately 8 spears) servings
Preparation time: 20 minutes
Chilling time: 8 hours

Nutrient Information (per serving):

Servings per recipe 6	Cholesterol <1 milligram
Serving size 8 asparagus spears	Sodium 130 milligrams
Carbohydrate choices 0	Dietary Fiber 2 grams
Calories 122	% calories from:
Carbohydrate 3 grams	Protein 16%
Protein 5 grams	Carbohydrate 10%
Fat 10 grams	Fat 74%
Saturated Fat 1 gram	

Food Exchanges: 1 vegetable, 2 fat

Chilled Cucumber Soup

A cool and refreshing start to a meal. Tangy, fresh-grated lemon rind and delicate-tasting chives complement the mildly flavored cucumber.

2 medium cucumbers
1/4 cup diced onion
1 cup water
1/8 teaspoon white pepper
1/4 teaspoon salt
1/4 cup all-purpose flour
2 cups reduced-sodium, fat-free chicken bouillon
3/4 cup fat-free sour cream
1 teaspoon grated lemon rind
1 tablespoon chopped fresh chives

Peel cucumbers and remove seeds. Slice and place in saucepan.

Add onion, water, pepper, and salt. Cook, uncovered, 25 minutes, or until cucumbers are very soft. Place contents of pan in food processor or blender and process until smooth. In separate pan stir together flour and 1/2 cup chicken bouillon to make a paste. Whisk in remaining bouillon and then cucumber purée. Place over low heat. When mixture begins to bubble, simmer for two minutes. Strain through sieve and chill at least two hours.

Just before serving stir in sour cream, lemon rind, and chives.

Makes 4 (1 cup) servings
Preparation time: 10 minutes
Cooking time: 30 minutes
Chilling time: 2 hours

Nutrient Information (per serving):

Servings per recipe 4	Cholesterol 0
Serving size 1 cup	Sodium 197 milligrams
Carbohydrate choices 1	Dietary Fiber 1 gram
Calories 89	% calories from:
Carbohydrate 13 grams	Protein 31%
Protein 7 grams	Carbohydrate 58%
Fat 1 gram	Fat 10%
Saturated Fat <1 gram	

Food Exchanges: 2 vegetable, 1/2 skim milk

Spicy Tortilla Chips

Munch alone, with the Quick Hummus Dip (page 37), or alongside the Chili Italiano (page 109)!

1½ Choices

S **F**

1/4 teaspoon garlic powder
1/4 teaspoon onion powder
1/2 teaspoon paprika
1/2 teaspoon salt
1/4 teaspoon black pepper
8 (8-inch) fat-free flour tortillas
Butter-flavored cooking spray
1 1/2 tablespoons corn oil

Preheat oven to 350°. In a small bowl mix together garlic powder, onion powder, paprika, salt, and pepper. Coat one side of each tortilla with cooking spray. Place tortillas sprayed-side down on baking sheet. Brush oil over tops of tortillas then sprinkle with seasoning mixture. Cut each tortilla into 6 wedges. Bake for 12 minutes, or until chips are crisp and edges are lightly browned and slightly curled. Serve warm or cooled.

Makes 8 (6 chip) servings
Preparation time: 10 minutes
Baking time: 12 minutes

Nutrient Information (per serving):

Servings per recipe 8	Cholesterol 0
Serving size 6 chips	Sodium 417 milligrams
Carbohydrate choices 1 1/2	Dietary Fiber 5 grams
Calories 112	% calories from:
Carbohydrate 17 grams	Protein 15%
Protein 3 grams	Carbohydrate 61%
Fat 3 grams	Fat 24%
Saturated Fat <1 gram	

Food Exchanges: 1 starch, 1 fat

Italian Artichoke Dip

*Serve in a hollowed-out round loaf of brown bread
with a sprig of parsley on top.*

0
Choices

1 cup reduced-fat sour cream

1/4 cup reduced-fat mayonnaise

1 packet dry Italian salad dressing mix

1 cup diced, canned artichoke hearts, rinsed and drained

In a medium bowl, mix together sour cream, mayonnaise, and salad dressing mix. Stir in artichoke hearts. Cover and chill at least 2 hours to allow flavors to blend.

Makes 14 (2 tablespoon) servings
Preparation time: 5 minutes
Chilling time: 2 hours

Nutrient Information (per serving):

Servings per recipe 14	Cholesterol 6 milligrams
Serving size 2 tablespoons	Sodium 249 milligrams
Carbohydrate choices 0	Dietary Fiber 0
Calories 51	% calories from:
Carbohydrate 4 grams	Protein 16%
Protein 2 grams	Carbohydrate 31%
Fat 3 grams	Fat 53%
Saturated Fat 1 gram	

Food Exchanges: 1 vegetable, 1/2 fat

Rich Broccoli and Cheese Dip

Serve with bagel crisps or low-fat snack crackers.

0 Choices

- 10 3/4-ounce can reduced-fat cream of mushroom soup
- 8 ounces fat-free processed cheese loaf, cut in cubes
- 14 1/2-ounce can tomatoes with green chilies
- 1 teaspoon garlic powder
- 1/8 teaspoon black pepper
- 4-ounce can sliced mushrooms, drained
- 2 10-ounce packages frozen chopped broccoli, thawed and drained

In a large saucepan, combine soup, cheese, tomatoes with green chilies, garlic powder, and black pepper. Warm over medium heat, stirring frequently, until cheese is melted and mixture is bubbly. Mix in mushrooms and broccoli and continue to heat for an additional 10 minutes, or until mixture is bubbly again.

Makes 32 (1/4 cup) servings
Preparation time: 20 minutes

Nutrient Information (per serving):

Servings per recipe 32	Cholesterol <1 milligram
Serving size 1/4 cup	Sodium 221 milligrams
Carbohydrate choices 0	Dietary Fiber 1 gram
Calories 21	% calories from:
Carbohydrate 2 grams	Protein 38%
Protein 2 grams	Carbohydrate 40%
Fat <1 gram	Fat 21%
Saturated Fat <1 gram	

Food Exchanges: Free

Great Gazpacho Dip

A great dip served with pita crisps or low-fat tortilla chips! You will find this dip reminiscent of the cold tomato and vegetable soup that is a popular summer fare.

0 Choices

- 4 Roma tomatoes, skin and seeds removed, finely chopped
- 1/2 yellow pepper, seeded and finely chopped
- 10 green onions, chopped
- 2 4 1/2-ounce cans chopped green chilies, drained
- 3 tablespoons corn oil
- 1/4 cup red wine vinegar
- 1/4 teaspoon crushed garlic
- 1/4 teaspoon salt
- 1/8 teaspoon black pepper

Place all ingredients in a large bowl and gently stir to combine. Cover and chill at least 4 hours to allow flavors to blend.

Note: The percentage of calories from fat in this dip appears high, but note that there are only 2 grams of fat per serving.

Makes 20 (1/4 cup) servings
Preparation time: 15 minutes
Chilling time: 4 hours

Nutrient Information (per serving):

Servings per recipe 20	Cholesterol 0
Serving size 1/4 cup	Sodium 75 milligrams
Carbohydrate choices 0	Dietary Fiber 1 gram
Calories 26	% calories from:
Carbohydrate 2 grams	Protein 0%
Protein <1 gram	Carbohydrate 31%
Fat 2 grams	Fat 69%
Saturated Fat <1 gram	

Food Exchanges: 1 vegetable

Quick Hummus Dip

Toasted pita bread triangles or our Spicy Tortilla Chips (page 33) make excellent accompaniments for this scrumptious dip.

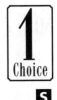

1 Choice

S

19-ounce can garbanzo beans, rinsed and drained

2 tablespoons tahini (sesame seed paste)

1/4 cup fresh lemon juice

2 tablespoons water

1 teaspoon salt

1 teaspoon crushed garlic

1/2 teaspoon ground cumin

1/8 teaspoon cayenne pepper

Place all ingredients in food processor and process until smooth. Best if chilled at least two hours to allow flavors to blend.

Makes 8 (1/4 cup) servings
Preparation time: 10 minutes
Chilling time: 2 hours

Nutrient Information (per serving):

Servings per recipe 8	Cholesterol 0
Serving size 1/4 cup	Sodium 439 milligrams
Carbohydrate choices 1	Dietary Fiber 3 grams
Calories 82	% calories from:
Carbohydrate 12 grams	Protein 20%
Protein 4 grams	Carbohydrate 59%
Fat 2 grams	Fat 22%
Saturated Fat <1 gram	

Food Exchanges: 1 starch

South-of-the-Border Dip

A speedy and spicy dip that will keep you coming back for more! Serve with your favorite baked tortilla chips.

1/2 Choice

31-ounce can fat-free refried beans
1 package taco seasoning mix
8 ounces fat-free sour cream
1 cup finely shredded reduced-fat cheddar cheese
1 cup mild salsa
2 cups chopped lettuce
2 tomatoes, seeded and finely diced

In a 2-quart microwavable serving dish, stir together beans and taco seasoning. Spread in bottom of dish and top with sour cream. Sprinkle with cheese, then microwave on High for 8 minutes, or until cheese melts and dip is hot in center. Remove from microwave and top with salsa, lettuce, and tomato (in that order).

Makes 28 (1/4 cup) servings
Preparation time: 10 minutes
Cooking time: 8 minutes

Nutrient Information (per serving):

Servings per recipe 28
Serving size 1/4 cup
Carbohydrate choices 1/2
Calories 53
Carbohydrate 7 grams
Protein 4 grams
Fat 1 gram
Saturated Fat <1 gram

Cholesterol 3 milligrams
Sodium 275 milligrams
Dietary Fiber 2 grams
% calories from:
   Protein 30%
   Carbohydrate 53%
   Fat 17%

Food Exchanges: 2 vegetable

Favorite Chipped Beef Spread

Always a favorite at get-togethers with family and friends!
Tastes best if made the night before to allow flavors to blend.
Serve on wheat crackers.

0 Choices

- 8 ounces fat-free cream cheese
- I teaspoon Worcestershire sauce
- I teaspoon skim milk
- 5 green onions, chopped
- 2 1/2-ounce package chipped beef, finely chopped

Place cream cheese in a large bowl and beat with an electric mixer until fluffy. Whip in Worcestershire sauce and milk. Stir in green onions and beef. Place in serving dish and refrigerate until serving time.

Makes 12 (2 tablespoon) servings
Preparation time: 5 minutes

Nutrient Information (per serving):

Servings per recipe 12	Cholesterol 5 milligrams
Serving size 2 tablespoons	Sodium 323 milligrams
Carbohydrate choices 0	Dietary Fiber <1 gram
Calories 25	% calories from:
Carbohydrate 1 gram	Protein 64%
Protein 4 grams	Carbohydrate 16%
Fat <1 gram	Fat 20%
Saturated Fat <1 gram	

Food Exchanges: 1 very lean meat

New England Crab Spread

Use a colorful baking dish for more eye-appeal.
Serve with assorted low-fat snack crackers.

4 ounces reduced-fat cream cheese
4 ounces fat-free cream cheese
2 tablespoons reduced-fat mayonnaise
2 tablespoons prepared horseradish
1/2 teaspoon lemon juice
1 tablespoon white cooking wine
1 tablespoon skim milk
6-ounce can white crab meat, drained and flaked
Cooking spray
Paprika

Preheat oven to 350°. Place cream cheeses, mayonnaise, and horseradish in a mixing bowl and whip until fluffy. Blend in lemon juice, wine, and milk. Stir in crab meat. Spread in baking dish coated with cooking spray and sprinkle lightly with paprika. Bake for 20 minutes or until bubbly.

Makes 16 (2 tablespoon) servings
Preparation time: 10 minutes
Baking time: 20 minutes

Nutrient Information (per serving):

Servings per recipe 16	Cholesterol 10 milligrams
Serving size 2 tablespoons	Sodium 145 milligrams
Carbohydrate choices 0	Dietary Fiber <1 gram
Calories 29	% calories from:
Carbohydrate 1 gram	Protein 55%
Protein 4 grams	Carbohydrate 14%
Fat 1 gram	Fat 31%
Saturated Fat <1 gram	

Food Exchanges: 1/2 very lean meat

Cocktail Chicken Spread

Serve this spread on party slices of rye or pumpernickel bread for a hit at your next festive occasion!

0 Choices

2 8-ounce packages fat-free cream cheese

1 tablespoon + 1 teaspoon A-1 steak sauce

2 cups boiled, finely minced chicken breast

5 green onions, finely chopped

1/3 cup minced celery

1/8 teaspoon salt

1/8 teaspoon coarse ground black pepper

Paprika

In a mixing bowl, combine cream cheese and steak sauce with an electric mixer, beating until fluffy. Blend in chicken, green onions, celery, salt, and pepper. Place in serving dish and chill overnight to allow flavors to blend.

Sprinkle lightly with paprika before serving.

Makes 21 (2 tablespoon) servings
Preparation time: 10 minutes
Chilling time: 8 hours

Nutrient Information (per serving):

Servings per recipe 21	Cholesterol 14 milligrams
Serving size 2 tablespoons	Sodium 174 milligrams
Carbohydrate choices 0	Dietary Fiber <1 gram
Calories 45	% calories from:
Carbohydrate 1 gram	Protein 71%
Protein 8 grams	Carbohydrate 9%
Fat 1 gram	Fat 20%
Saturated Fat <1 gram	

Food Exchanges: 1 very lean meat

Mini Pita Pizzas

Pita bread makes a quick and easy crust for these pizzas!

1½ Choices

4 (6-inch) pita bread rounds
1/2 cup pizza sauce
4 Roma tomatoes, thinly sliced
1/4 teaspoon crushed dried oregano
1/2 teaspoon dried basil
1 cup thinly sliced fresh mushrooms
4 thin slices purple onion, separated into rings
1 cup (4 ounces) shredded part-skim mozzarella cheese
2 tablespoons grated fat-free Parmesan cheese

Preheat oven to 350°. Place pita bread rounds on an ungreased baking sheet and warm in oven for 10 minutes. Remove from oven and spread top of each pita round with 2 tablespoons pizza sauce, leaving a 1/2-inch border. Top pita rounds with tomato slices. Sprinkle with oregano and basil. Arrange mushrooms and onion over tomato. Sprinkle with mozzarella, then Parmesan cheese. Increase oven temperature to broil. Place pizzas in oven 5 inches from heat source and leave oven door partially open. Broil for 4 minutes, or until cheese melts and pizzas are thoroughly heated. Cut each round into 4 wedges.

Makes 8 (2 wedge) servings
Preparation time: 10 minutes
Cooking time: 14 minutes

Nutrient Information (per serving):

Servings per recipe 8

Serving size 2 wedges

Carbohydrate choices 1 1/2

Calories 147

Carbohydrate 22 grams

Protein 8 grams

Fat 3 grams

Saturated Fat 2 grams

Cholesterol 8 milligrams

Sodium 363 milligrams

Dietary Fiber 1 gram

% calories from:

Protein 22 %

Carbohydrate 60 %

Fat 18 %

Food Exchanges: 1/2 starch, 1 low-fat milk

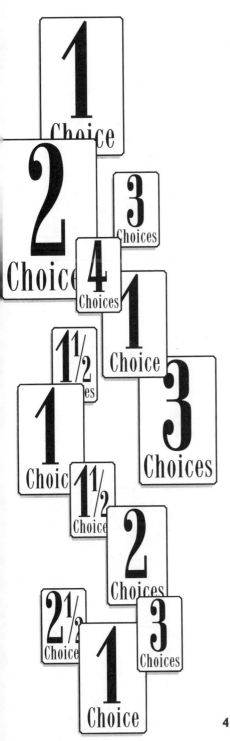

Breads

Broccoli Cheese Bread

This colorful variation on traditional corn bread is a nice accompaniment to the Navy Bean and Ham Soup (page 131).

S

1 cup liquid egg substitute

1/2 cup water

4 tablespoons reduced-calorie margarine, melted

1 teaspoon salt

2 cups corn bread mix

10-ounce package frozen chopped broccoli, thawed and drained

1 large onion, finely diced

1 cup shredded reduced-fat cheddar cheese

Cooking spray

Preheat oven to 400°. In a bowl, mix together the first 5 ingredients. Stir in the broccoli, onion, and cheese. Spoon into a 9" x 13" baking pan coated with cooking spray and bake for 25 minutes, or until toothpick inserted in center of bread comes out clean. Serve warm.

Makes 15 (1 square) servings
Preparation time: 10 minutes
Baking time: 25 minutes

Nutrient Information (per serving):

Servings per recipe 15

Serving size 1 square

Carbohydrate choices 1 1/2

Calories 128

Carbohydrate 16 grams

Protein 7 grams

Fat 4 grams

Saturated Fat 1 gram

Cholesterol 6 milligrams

Sodium 517 milligrams

Dietary Fiber 1 gram

% calories from:

Protein 22%

Carbohydrate 50%

Fat 28%

Food Exchanges: 1 starch, 1 lean meat

Garlic Parmesan Pull-Apart Bread

"There are many miracles in the world to be celebrated and, for me, garlic is the most deserving."—Leo Buscaglia. Celebrate the flavor of garlic in this innovative version of garlic bread!

> 5 tablespoons reduced-calorie stick margarine, melted
> I teaspoon garlic salt
> 1/4 teaspoon garlic powder
> I 1/2 teaspoons dried dillweed
> I teaspoon crushed dried oregano
> 25-ounce package frozen roll dough, thawed
> 5 tablespoons grated Parmesan cheese
> Cooking spray

In a small bowl, combine melted margarine, garlic salt, garlic powder, dill, and oregano. Place Parmesan cheese in a separate small bowl. Dip dough balls in margarine mixture and then roll in Parmesan cheese to lightly coat. Arrange in a Bundt pan coated well with cooking spray. Lay wax paper across the top of the pan and set in a warm place to rise for 4 hours, or until dough fills pan (may also prepare in the morning using unthawed roll dough and let rise 8 hours during the day). Preheat oven to 350°. Bake for 30 minutes, or until golden.

Makes 14 servings
Preparation time: 10 minutes
Rising time: 4 hours
Baking time: 30 minutes

Nutrient Information (per serving):

Servings per recipe 14

Serving size 1 1/2 bread balls

Carbohydrate choices 2

Calories 181

Carbohydrate 29 grams

Protein 5 grams

Fat 5 grams

Saturated Fat 2 grams

Cholesterol 4 milligrams

Sodium 518 milligrams

Dietary Fiber 1 gram

% calories from:

Protein 11%

Carbohydrate 64%

Fat 25%

Food Exchanges: 2 starch, 1 fat

Berry Patch Muffins

These muffins can be made any time of year since they use frozen blackberries instead of fresh.

2 1/2 cups all-purpose flour

1/2 teaspoon baking soda

2 teaspoons baking powder

1/4 teaspoon salt

1/2 cup brown sugar

1 1/2 cups low-fat buttermilk

1/4 cup corn oil

1 egg

1/2 teaspoon lemon extract

1 teaspoon vanilla extract

1/2 teaspoon butter flavoring

12-ounce package frozen, unsweetened blackberries, thawed

Cooking spray

Preheat oven to 350°. Place flour, baking soda, baking powder, salt, and brown sugar in a large bowl. Stir to combine and then make a well in center of mixture.

In a separate bowl, mix together buttermilk, oil, egg, extracts, and butter flavoring. Add to flour mixture and stir until dry ingredients are just moistened. Gently stir in blackberries (rinse berries first if juicy; take care not to stir too much or dough will turn blue). Spoon batter into 20 muffin cups coated with cooking spray, filling cups 3/4 full. Bake for 23 minutes or until muffins spring back when touched.

Makes 20 (1 muffin) servings
Preparation time: 15 minutes
Baking time: 23 minutes

Nutrient Information (per serving):

Servings per recipe 20	Cholesterol 11 milligrams
Serving size 1 muffin	Sodium 132 milligrams
Carbohydrate choices 1 1/2	Dietary Fiber 2 grams
Calories 115	% calories from:
Carbohydrate 19 grams	Protein 10%
Protein 3 grams	Carbohydrate 66%
Fat 3 grams	Fat 23%
Saturated Fat 1 gram	

Food Exchanges: 1 starch, 1 fat

Ready-in-a-Flash Rolls

"Bread is like dresses, hats, and shoes—in other words, essential!"—Emily Post

2 cups self-rising flour
1 1/2 teaspoons sugar
1 cup skim milk
5 tablespoons low-fat mayonnaise
Cooking spray

Preheat oven to 450°. Place all ingredients in a bowl and stir until combined. Spoon into muffin tins coated with cooking spray. Bake for 13 minutes, or until golden.

Makes 12 (1 roll) servings
Preparation time: 5 minutes
Baking time: 13 minutes

Nutrient Information (per serving):

Servings per recipe 12
Serving size 1 roll
Carbohydrate choices 1 1/2
Calories 98
Carbohydrate 17 grams
Protein 3 grams
Fat 2 grams
Saturated Fat <1 gram

Cholesterol 2 milligrams
Sodium 281 milligrams
Dietary Fiber 3 grams
% calories from:
Protein 12%
Carbohydrate 69%
Fat 18%

Food Exchanges: 1 starch, 1/2 fat

Pumpkin Spice Muffins

The array of spices in this moist muffin provides a harmony of flavors and enhanced sweetness.

1 1/2
Choices

1 1/2 cups all-purpose flour
1/2 cup whole wheat flour
1 1/2 teaspoons baking powder
1/2 teaspoon baking soda
1 1/2 teaspoons cinnamon
1/8 teaspoon ground cloves
1/2 teaspoon ground nutmeg
1/2 teaspoon allspice
3/4 cup brown sugar
1 cup canned pumpkin
1/4 cup liquid egg substitute
1/3 cup skim milk
1/4 cup corn oil
3 ounces frozen unsweetened orange juice concentrate, thawed
Cooking spray

Preheat oven to 400°. In a large bowl, sift together flours, baking powder, baking soda, cinnamon, cloves, nutmeg, and allspice. Stir in brown sugar. In a separate bowl combine pumpkin, egg substitute, milk, oil, and orange juice concentrate; stir together. Add wet ingredients to dry ingredients, stirring until just moistened. Spoon into 18 muffin cups coated with cooking spray and bake for 14 minutes.

Makes 18 (1 muffin) servings
Preparation time: 10 minutes
Baking time: 14 minutes

Nutrient Information (per serving):

Servings per recipe 18

Serving size 1 muffin

Carbohydrate choices 1 1/2

Calories 127

Carbohydrate 23 grams

Protein 2 grams

Fat 3 grams

Saturated Fat <1 gram

Cholesterol <1 milligram

Sodium 89 milligrams

Dietary Fiber 1 gram

% calories from:

Protein 6%

Carbohydrate 72%

Fat 21%

Food Exchanges: 1/2 starch, 1 fruit, 1 fat

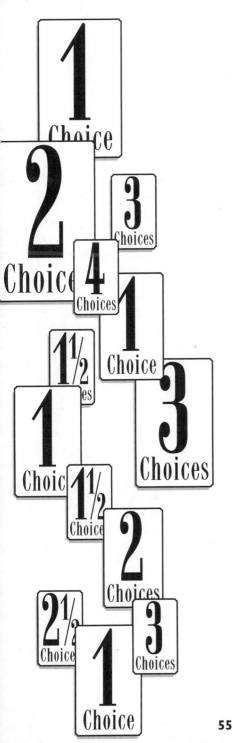

Salads

Spaghetti Salad Supreme

This is a great salad for cookouts! Flavor improves if it is refrigerated for a couple of hours before serving.

S

- 1 pound spaghetti, cooked according to package directions
- 3 Roma tomatoes, seeded and diced
- 1 green pepper, seeded and diced
- 1 cucumber, peeled, seeded, and diced
- 1 medium purple onion, diced
- 8-ounce package mushrooms, sliced
- 8-ounce bottle reduced-fat Italian dressing
- 1/2 cup plus 2 tablespoons McCormick's Salad Supreme (usually found in spice section)

Place all ingredients in a large serving dish and toss well.

Makes 12 (1 cup) servings
Preparation time: 20 minutes

Nutrient Information (per serving):

Servings per recipe 12
Serving size 1 cup
Carbohydrate choices 2 1/2
Calories 183
Carbohydrate 33 grams
Protein 6 grams
Fat 3 grams
Saturated Fat <1 gram

Cholesterol 1 milligram
Sodium 863 milligrams
Dietary Fiber 1 gram
% calories from:
   Protein 13%
   Carbohydrate 72%
   Fat 15%

Food Exchanges: 2 starch, 1 vegetable

Colorful Ranch-Style Salad

This colorful salad is packed with flavor and good nutrition. Best if chilled overnight to allow flavors to blend.

8 ounces fresh carrots, peeled and sliced
3 cups fresh bite-size cauliflower florets
3 cups fresh bite-size broccoli florets
1/2 cup reduced-fat ranch-style salad dressing

Combine vegetables in a large bowl. Add dressing and toss to coat. Cover and refrigerate 8 hours, or overnight, for best flavor.

Makes 15 (1/2 cup) servings
Preparation time: 15 minutes
Chilling time: 8 hours

Nutrient Information (per serving):

Servings per recipe 15
Serving size 1/2 cup
Carbohydrate choices 0
Calories 42
Carbohydrate 4 grams
Protein 2 grams
Fat 2 grams
Saturated Fat <1 gram

Cholesterol 0
Sodium 109 milligrams
Dietary Fiber 2 grams
% calories from:
  Protein 19%
  Carbohydrate 38%
  Fat 43%

Food Exchanges: 1 vegetable, 1/2 fat

Herbed Tomato Slices

A quick and refreshing old-fashioned salad. The robust flavor of oregano complements the tanginess of fresh, juicy tomatoes.

6 medium tomatoes, sliced

2 1/2 tablespoons red wine vinegar

1 1/2 tablespoons canola oil

1/2 teaspoon salt

1/4 teaspoon sugar

1/4 teaspoon black pepper

3/4 teaspoon crushed dried oregano

Layer tomato slices in shallow serving dish. Place vinegar, oil, salt, sugar, pepper, and oregano in a jar. Cover tightly with lid and shake to combine. Pour dressing over tomatoes and chill in refrigerator for 2 hours.

Makes 6 (1 tomato) servings
Preparation time: 10 minutes
Chilling time: 2 hours

Nutrient Information (per serving):

Servings per recipe 6	Cholesterol 0
Serving size 1 sliced tomato	Sodium 138 milligrams
Carbohydrate choices 1/2	Dietary Fiber <1 gram
Calories 51	% calories from:
Carbohydrate 5 grams	Protein 8%
Protein 1 gram	Carbohydrate 39%
Fat 3 grams	Fat 53%
Saturated Fat <1 gram	

Food Exchanges: 1 vegetable, 1/2 fat

Overnight Marinated Vegetable Salad

0 Choices

The broccoli, cauliflower, and asparagus are lightly steamed in this recipe to add tenderness, yet preserve nutrients. Savor the flavorful marinade that gently coats this colorful array of vegetables. Shorten the preparation time by using broccoli, cauliflower, and carrots purchased from the supermarket salad bar.

Salad:

3 cups bite-size broccoli florets

3 cups bite-size cauliflower florets

1/2 pound asparagus, each stalk cut in 3 slices on the diagonal

1 carrot, peeled and shredded

1 cucumber, peeled and cubed

1 zucchini, julienne sliced

15 cherry tomatoes, halved

Marinade:

5 tablespoons canola oil

2 tablespoons olive oil

3 tablespoons white wine vinegar

2 1/2 tablespoons fresh squeezed lemon juice

1 teaspoon Worcestershire sauce

1/8 teaspoon Tabasco sauce

1 teaspoon minced garlic

1 teaspoon grated onion

1/2 teaspoon black pepper

1/4 teaspoon salt

Place broccoli and cauliflower in a covered steamer pan over 2 inches boiling water for 5 minutes, or until crisp-tender. Run under cold water, drain, and set aside. Repeat this procedure with the asparagus, steaming the asparagus only 3 minutes, or until it just turns bright green.

Place all marinade ingredients in a large jar and shake well.

Combine all vegetables in a large zip-top plastic bag (may need 2 bags) and add marinade. Fasten the bag(s) tightly and gently turn until the vegetables are evenly coated. Refrigerate salad overnight, or 8 hours, turning the bag(s) once or twice.

Makes 14 (1 cup) servings
Preparation time: 35 minutes
Chilling time: 8 hours

Nutrient Information (per serving):

Servings per recipe 14	Cholesterol 0
Serving size 1 cup	Sodium 62 milligrams
Carbohydrate choices 0	Dietary Fiber 3 grams
Calories 73	% calories from:
Carbohydrate 4 grams	Protein 16%
Protein 3 grams	Carbohydrate 22%
Fat 5 grams	Fat 62%
Saturated Fat <1 gram	

Food Exchanges: 1 vegetable, 1 fat

Snappy Snow Pea Salad

Fresh, crispy, and colorful! Buy sliced mushrooms and shredded carrots off the supermarket salad bar to make preparation even quicker.

S

3 cups fresh snow peas in pods, strings removed
8-ounce can sliced water chestnuts, drained
1 cup thinly sliced fresh mushrooms
1/4 cup shredded carrot
3 tablespoons reduced-sodium soy sauce
6 tablespoons rice wine vinegar
1/2 teaspoon garlic powder
1/4 teaspoon ground ginger

Place snow peas in a steamer basket, cover, and steam over 2 inches boiling water for 3 minutes. Remove from heat and run under cold water to stop the cooking process. In a large serving dish, combine snow peas and remaing vegetables.

Combine soy sauce, vinegar, garlic powder, and ginger in a jar. Cover tightly with lid and shake to combine. Pour vinegar mixture over snow pea mixture and toss to coat. Chill for at least 1 hour to allow flavors to blend.

Makes 5 (1 cup) servings
Preparation time: 15 minutes
Chilling time: 1 hour

Nutrient Information (per serving):

Servings per recipe 5	Cholesterol 0
Serving size 1 cup	Sodium 517 milligrams
Carbohydrate choices 1 1/2	Dietary Fiber 3 grams
Calories 85	% calories from:
Carbohydrate 16 grams	Protein 19%
Protein 4 grams	Carbohydrate 75%
Fat <1 gram	Fat 6%
Saturated Fat <1 gram	

Food Exchanges: 3 vegetable

Crispy Cucumbers and Onions

1/2 Choice

This is an old favorite family recipe that has been passed down from Tami's grandmother. It is a light and refreshing addition to a summer meal from the grill, be it pork chops, chicken breasts, or hamburgers.

- 2 cups water
- 1 cup white vinegar
- 3/4 teaspoon salt
- 2 cucumbers, peeled and sliced
- 1 large onion, sliced and separated into rings

In a deep container with a lid, stir together water, vinegar, and salt. Add cucumbers and onions, then cover tightly with lid. Place in refrigerator and chill 3 hours or longer to allow flavors to blend. Drain before serving.

Makes 6 (1 cup) servings
Preparation time: 10 minutes
Chilling time: 3 hours

Nutrient Information (per serving):

Servings per recipe 6	Cholesterol 0
Serving size 1 cup	Sodium 57 milligrams
Carbohydrate choices 1/2	Dietary Fiber 1 gram
Calories 33	% calories from:
Carbohydrate 6 grams	Protein 12%
Protein 1 gram	Carbohydrate 73%
Fat <1 gram	Fat 15%
Saturated Fat <1 gram	

Food Exchanges: 1 vegetable

Chinese Sprout Salad

1/2 Choice

For a melding of flavors, the dressing may be prepared ahead and stored in the refrigerator until time to toss with this crunchy salad.

Salad:

4 cups Boston red leaf lettuce

3/4 cup bean sprouts, rinsed and drained

1/2 dup diced water chestnuts, rinsed and drained

1/2 cup finely chopped green onions

2 tablespoons toasted sesame seeds

Dressing:

1 cup fat-free sour cream

2 tablespoons reduced-fat mayonnaise

2 tablespoons skim milk

1 tablespoon reduced-sodium soy sauce

1/4 teaspoon ground ginger

2 tablespoons chopped, dried parsley

Combine salad ingredients in large salad bowl and set aside. Combine dressing ingredients in separate bowl and mix well using a wire whisk. Pour dressing over salad and toss to coat.

Makes 6 (1 cup) servings
Preparation time: 10 minutes

Nutrient Information (per serving):

Servings per recipe 6	Cholesterol 2 milligrams
Serving size 1 cup	Sodium 202 milligrams
Carbohydrate choices 1/2	Dietary Fiber 1 gram
Calories 79	% calories from:
Carbohydrate 7 grams	Protein 30%
Protein 6 grams	Carbohydrate 35%
Fat 3 grams	Fat 34%
Saturated Fat <1 gram	

Food Exchanges: 1 vegetable, 1 fat

Cinnamon Apple-Raisin Slaw

A sweet and crunchy salad. Shorten the preparation time by buying a 16-ounce bag pre-shredded cabbage at the supermarket.

1
Choice

16-ounce bag rainbow salad (broccoli, cauliflower, carrots, and red cabbage) or 1 large head cabbage, finely shredded

2 red apples, chopped into bite-size chunks

1/2 cup golden raisins

3 tablespoons corn oil

3 tablespoons apple cider vinegar

2 teaspoons honey

1 teaspoon ground cinnamon

In a large bowl, combine rainbow salad, apple, and raisins. In a small bowl, whisk together oil, vinegar, honey, and cinnamon. Drizzle over cabbage mixture and toss to coat. Chill 1 hour.

Makes 14 (1/2 cup) servings
Preparation time: 15 minutes
Chilling time: 1 hour

Nutrient Information (per serving):

Servings per recipe 14	Cholesterol 0
Serving size 1/2 cup	Sodium 7 milligrams
Carbohydrate choices 1	Dietary Fiber 1 gram
Calories 67	% calories from:
Carbohydrate 9 grams	Protein 6%
Protein 1 gram	Carbohydrate 54%
Fat 3 grams	Fat 40%
Saturated Fat <1 gram	

Food Exchanges: 1 vegetable, 1 fat

Greco-Italian Tossed Salad

A riot of flavors and color spring forth from this salad! The tangy tomato vinaigrette dressing contributes a significant amount of fat, so enjoy salad alongside a main dish low in fat.

Pita Croutons:

1 tablespoon canola oil

1/8 teaspoon garlic salt

1/4 teaspoon crushed dried oregano

1 (8-inch) round pita bread sliced in half to form two circles

Tomato Vinaigrette:

2 Roma tomatoes, skin and seeds removed

2 tablespoons white wine vinegar

1 teaspoon chopped fresh basil (or 1/2 teaspoon dried basil)

1/2 teaspoon salt

1/8 teaspoon coarse ground black pepper

1/4 cup canola oil

Salad:

1 head red leaf lettuce

1/2 small purple onion, sliced and separated into rings

2 ounces feta cheese, crumbled

To prepare croutons, preheat oven to 400°. Combine oil, garlic salt, and oregano in a small bowl; stir well. Brush oil mixture over both sides of each pita circle. Cut each pita circle into bite-size triangles and place on a baking sheet. Bake for 7 minutes, or until croutons are light golden and crisp. Cool.

To prepare vinaigrette, purée the tomato in a food processor. Add vinegar, basil, salt, pepper, and half the oil. Process. Add remaining oil and process again. Place in the refrigerator to chill while preparing the salad. Vinaigrette can be made 2 to 3 days in advance if desired.

Remove and discard the vein from each lettuce leaf, then tear lettuce into bite-size pieces and place in a large salad bowl. Lay onion rings over lettuce. Sprinkle with cheese.

Before serving, add croutons to salad, drizzle with tomato vinaigrette, and toss to coat.

Makes 7 (2 cup) servings
Preparation time: 30 minutes

Nutrient Information (per serving):

Servings per recipe 7

Serving size 2 cups

Carbohydrate choices 1

Calories 168

Carbohydrate 12 grams

Protein 3 grams

Fat 12 grams

Saturated Fat 2 grams

Cholesterol 7 milligrams

Sodium 338 milligrams

Dietary Fiber <1 gram

% calories from:

  Protein 7%

  Carbohydrate 29%

  Fat 64%

Food Exchanges: 2 1/2 vegetable, 2 fat

Picante Red-Skin Potato Salad

Choice

Potato salad has been a fundamental food in households across America since its popularity arose in the late 1800s. The red potato skins add color and fiber to this salad, which uses picante sauce in place of the traditional mayonnaise.

2 pounds red-skin potatoes
2 slices turkey bacon, cooked, drained, and crumbled
1 cup finely diced celery
1/4 cup finely diced green onions
1/2 cup medium picante sauce
1/4 cup reduced-fat sour cream
1/4 teaspoon salt
1/2 teaspoon ground cumin

Place potatoes in a large pan, cover with water, and cook over medium heat for 20 minutes, or until potatoes are tender when pierced with a fork. Drain and cool potatoes, dice into bite-size cubes, then place in a large bowl. Add turkey bacon, celery, and onion to potatoes. Set aside.

In a separate bowl, stir together picante sauce, sour cream, salt, and ground cumin. Add to potato mixture and toss to coat. Cover and chill at least 1 hour or until serving time.

Makes 16 (1/2 cup) servings
Preparation time: 15 minutes
Cooking time: 20 minutes
Chilling time: 1 hour

Nutrient Information (per serving):

Servings per recipe 16

Serving size 1/2 cup

Carbohydrate choices 1

Calories 57

Carbohydrate 10 grams

Protein 2 grams

Fat 1 gram

Saturated Fat <1 gram

Cholesterol 3 milligrams

Sodium 121 milligrams

Dietary Fiber 1 gram

% calories from:

Protein 14%

Carbohydrate 70%

Fat 16%

Food Exchanges: 1 starch

Strawberry Spinach Salad with Toasted Almonds

$\frac{1}{2}$
Choice

F

You'll find that the strawberries' sweetness offsets the somewhat sharp flavor of the spinach. The end result—a charming flavor combination!

Dressing:

2 tablespoons canola oil

1/4 cup red wine vinegar

2 packets saccharin sweetener

1/4 teaspoon salt

1/8 teaspoon black pepper

1/4 teaspoon garlic powder

1/4 teaspoon onion powder

1/4 teaspoon dry mustard

Salad:

10-ounce package fresh spinach, washed, drained, and stems removed

2 cups sliced fresh strawberries

1/4 cup sliced almonds, lightly toasted

Place dressing ingredients in a jar. Cover tightly with lid and shake to combine. Refrigerate at least 1 hour to allow flavors to blend.

In a large salad bowl, combine spinach, strawberries, and almonds. Pour dressing over salad and toss to coat.

Note: To decrease the fat content of this salad, the almonds can be omitted.

Makes 6 (1 cup) servings
Preparation time: 15 minutes
Chilling time: 1 hour

Nutrient Information (per serving):

Servings per recipe 6

Serving size 1 cup

Carbohydrate choices 1/2

Calories 95

Carbohydrate 5 grams

Protein 3 grams

Fat 7 grams

Saturated Fat <1 gram

Cholesterol 0

Sodium 148 milligrams

Dietary Fiber 5 grams

% calories from:

Protein 13%

Carbohydrate 21%

Fat 66%

Food Exchanges: 1 vegetable, 1 1/2 fat

Oriental Chicken Salad

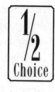

Fresh-squeezed lemon juice adds a zip to this chicken salad that's full of crunch. For a unique serving "dish," slice off the top of a large tomato, hollow it out, stuff with Oriental Chicken Salad, and top with a green pepper "lid" (the top of a green pepper).

- 4 cups shredded boiled chicken breast
- 8-ounce can sliced water chestnuts, drained and chopped
- 3 green onions, diced
- 1/4 cup unsalted peanuts, chopped
- 1 tablespoon + 1 teaspoon reduced-sodium soy sauce
- 1 teaspoon fresh-squeezed lemon juice
- 1/2 teaspoon coarse ground black pepper
- 3/4 cup reduced-fat mayonnaise

Place chicken, water chestnuts, green onions, and peanuts in a large bowl. Set aside. In a separate bowl, stir together soy sauce, lemon juice, pepper, and mayonnaise. Add to chicken mixture and toss to coat. Cover and refrigerate at least 1 hour to allow flavors to blend.

Makes 8 (1/2 cup) servings
Preparation time: 15 minutes
Chilling time: 1 hour

Nutrient Information (per serving):

Servings per recipe 8
Serving size 1/2 cup
Carbohydrate choices 1/2
Calories 301
Carbohydrate 6 grams
Protein 31 grams
Fat 17 grams
Saturated Fat 4 grams

Cholesterol 83 milligrams
Sodium 340 milligrams
Dietary Fiber 2 grams
% calories from:
  Protein 41%
  Carbohydrate 8%
  Fat 51%

Food Exchanges: 1 vegetable, 4 lean meat, 1 fat

Spicy Southwestern Bean Salad

For an extra special touch, serve this salad in red or yellow peppers that have the tops sliced off and seeds removed.

1 tablespoon corn oil

Cooking spray

2 tablespoons chopped pickled jalapeno pepper

1 teaspoon crushed garlic

1 teaspoon ground cumin

15-ounce can black-eyed peas, rinsed and drained

15 1/2-ounce can black beans, rinsed and drained

2 green onions, finely chopped

1 tablespoon chopped fresh parsley

1/4 teaspoon salt

3 Roma tomatoes, seeded and diced

Put corn oil in large nonstick skillet coated with cooking spray and place over medium heat. Add pepper, garlic, and cumin. Cook, uncovered, for 3 minutes, stirring periodically. Remove from heat. Add black-eyed peas, black beans, onions, parsley, and salt. Toss to combine. Place in serving dish, cover, and refrigerate 8 hours, or overnight, to allow flavors to blend.

Before serving, toss in tomato.

Makes 7 (1/2 cup) servings
Preparation time: 10 minutes
Chilling time: 8 hours

Nutrient Information (per serving):

Servings per recipe 7
Serving size 1/2 cup
Carbohydrate choices 1 1/2
Calories 147
Carbohydrate 22 grams
Protein 8 grams
Fat 3 grams
Saturated Fat <1 gram

Cholesterol 0
Sodium 119 milligrams
Dietary Fiber 8 grams
% calories from:
  Protein 22%
  Carbohydrate 60%
  Fat 18%

Food Exchanges: 1 1/2 starch, 1 vegetable

Creamy Orange Gelatin

Gelatin salads can be tricky to unmold. Try these tips: To loosen the gelatin, moisten tips of clean fingers with water and gently pull gelatin from edge of mold. Dipping the mold in warm water for 10 seconds (just up to the rim of the mold) further enables the gelatin to unmold easily.

0.3-ounce package sugar-free orange gelatin

1 1/2 cups boiling water

8 ounces fat-free cream cheese

1/4 cup orange juice

1 tablespoon lemon juice

1 tablespoon fresh grated orange rind

Place gelatin in a large bowl. Add boiling water and stir until gelatin is dissolved. In a separate bowl, beat cream cheese with an electric mixer until fluffy. Add gelatin to cream cheese and beat until combined. Whip in orange juice, lemon juice, and orange rind. Pour into 1-quart gelatin mold and chill until firm, or about 1 hour. Unmold and serve.

Makes 6 (1 cup) servings
Preparation time: 10 minutes
Chilling time: 1 hour

Nutrient Information (per serving):

Servings per recipe 6	Cholesterol 0
Serving size 1 cup	Sodium 257 milligrams
Carbohydrate choices 0	Dietary Fiber <1 gram
Calories 41	% calories from:
Carbohydrate 3 grams	Protein 59%
Protein 6 grams	Carbohydrate 29%
Fat <1 gram	Fat 12%
Saturated Fat <1 gram	

Food Exchanges: 1 very lean meat

Pineapple Jubilee

2½
Choices

A jubilee of flavors that can be served on a lettuce leaf as a salad or in a sherbet cup as a dessert.

1 cup sugar-free vanilla yogurt
2 tablespoons frozen orange juice concentrate, thawed
2 15 1/4-ounce cans juice-packed pineapple chunks, drained
1/4 cup golden raisins
1/4 cup diced maraschino cherries, rinsed and drained
1/4 cup finely chopped walnuts

Combine yogurt and orange juice concentrate in a large bowl. Stir in pineapple, raisins, cherries, and walnuts. Chill 30 minutes. Serve using a slotted spoon.

Makes 5 (1 cup) servings
Preparation time: 5 minutes
Chilling time: 30 minutes

Nutrient Information (per serving):

Servings per recipe 5
Serving size 1 cup
Carbohydrate choices 2 1/2
Calories 188
Carbohydrate 33 grams
Protein 5 grams
Fat 4 grams
Saturated Fat <1 gram

Cholesterol 0
Sodium 24 milligrams
Dietary Fiber 2 grams
% calories from:
  Protein 11%
  Carbohydrate 70%
  Fat 19%

Food Exchanges: 1 1/2 fruit, 1 skim milk

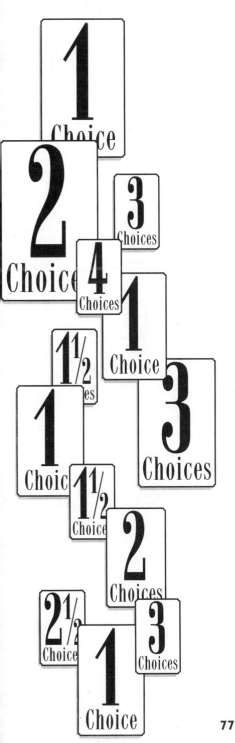

Entrées

Tender Pork Chops with Mushroom Gravy

Mouth-watering pork chops nestled in rich-tasting mushroom gravy. So tender you can cut them with a fork. Crockpot cooking at its best!

- 1/2 cup all-purpose flour
- 1 1/2 teaspoons dry ground mustard
- 1/8 teaspoon black pepper
- 1/2 teaspoon salt
- 1/2 teaspoon garlic powder
- 6 (1-inch thick) lean pork loin chops, fat trimmed
- Cooking spray
- 16-ounce can reduced-sodium, fat-free chicken broth
- 7-ounce can sliced mushrooms, drained

Preheat Crockpot on high. In a shallow dish, combine flour, mustard, pepper, salt, and garlic powder. Coat chops with flour mixture and place in nonstick skillet coated with cooking spray. Cook over medium-high heat until both sides of chops are browned, about 3 minutes per side.

While chops are browning, whisk together remaining flour mixture and chicken broth in Crockpot. When chops are browned, add to crockpot, along with mushrooms. Cook, covered, on high for 2 1/2 hours, or until tender. Stir periodically throughout cooking.

Makes 6 (1 chop, 1/4 cup gravy) servings
Preparation time: 10 minutes
Cooking time: 2 1/2 hours

Nutrient Information (per serving):

Servings per recipe 6

Serving size 1 chop with 1/4 c. gravy

Carbohydrate choices 1

Calories 203

Carbohydrate 10 grams

Protein 25 grams

Fat 7 grams

Saturated Fat 2 grams

Cholesterol 62 milligrams

Sodium 415 milligrams

Dietary Fiber 1 gram

% calories from:

   Protein 49%

   Carbohydrate 20%

   Fat 31%

Food Exchanges: 1 starch, 3 lean meat

Chinese Pepper Pork

The rice sticks used in this dish are a type of thin noodle made from rice. Find them in the oriental section of your supermarket.

   1 1/2 tablespoons sesame oil

   Cooking spray

   3/4 cup all-purpose flour

   1 teaspoon salt

   1/2 teaspoon black pepper

   1/2 teaspoon garlic powder

   1 1/2 pounds pork loin, cut in 1-inch cubes

   3 tablespoons Worcestershire sauce

   1 1/2 tablespoons reduced-sodium soy sauce

   2 cups water

   1/2 green pepper, seeded and cut in strips

   1/2 red pepper, seeded and cut in strips

   1 large onion, cut in rings and separated

   2 cups sliced fresh mushrooms

   8-ounce package rice sticks, cooked according to package
      directions

Place sesame oil in a nonstick skillet coated with cooking spray and warm over medium heat. Meanwhile, in a zip-top plastic bag, combine flour, salt, black pepper, and garlic powder. Add meat to bag, zip closed, and shake to coat. Place coated meat and remaining flour mixture in hot oil and cook over medium heat until meat is browned. Drain off any fat. Add Worcestershire sauce, soy sauce, and water to meat, cover pan, and simmer for 15 minutes, or until meat is tender; stir periodically (mixture will be thick). Add green and red peppers, onion, and mushrooms. Cover and continue cooking for 15 minutes, stirring periodically. May thin meat mixture with additional water if desired. Toss meat mixture with cooked rice sticks.

Makes 4 (1 cup sauce, 1 3/4 cup rice sticks) servings
Preparation time: 15 minutes
Cooking time: 30 minutes

Nutrient Information (per serving):

Servings per recipe 4	Cholesterol 134 milligrams
Serving size 1 cup sauce, 1 3/4 cups rice sticks	Sodium 1641 milligrams
	Dietary Fiber 3 grams
Carbohydrate choices 4	% calories from:
Calories 570	Protein 39%
Carbohydrate 55 grams	Carbohydrate 39%
Protein 56 grams	Fat 21%
Fat 14 grams	
Saturated Fat 4 grams	

Food Exchanges: 3 starch, 1 vegetable, 6 lean meat

Teriyaki Pork Kabobs

A colorful meal on a stick! Kabobs may be prepared ahead and stored in the refrigerator until grilling time. Delicious served with a baked potato or rice.

Choice

S

Marinade:
I cup reduced-sodium soy sauce
1/4 cup cooking sherry
I teaspoon minced garlic
1/8 teaspoon ginger
I teaspoon sugar

I pound boneless pork loin chops, cut into 16 cubes
2 medium zucchini, cut in 16 1/2-inch thick slices
2 purple onions, each cut into 8 sections
16 cherry tomatoes
2 large yellow peppers, seeded and each cut into 8 sections
16 whole fresh mushrooms

Place marinade ingredients in a jar with a lid. Put lid on tightly and shake to combine. Pour marinade into zip-top plastic bag, add pork cubes, close bag securely, and place in refrigerator for 8 hours or overnight. Shake bag periodically to coat meat.

Drain marinade, reserving it for basting. On each of 8 skewers, arrange 1 cube pork, followed by 1 slice zucchini, 1 section onion, 1 cherry tomato, 1 section pepper, and 1 mushroom. Repeat layering again on each skewer ending with a mushroom. Grill kabobs over medium heat for 20 minutes, or until pork is tender and no longer pink. Baste pork and vegetables twice during first 5 minutes of cooking and then discard remainder of marinade.

Makes 8 (I kabob) servings
Preparation time: 30 minutes
Chilling time: 8 hours
Cooking time: 20 minutes

Nutrient Information (per serving):

Servings per recipe 8

Serving size 1 kabob

Carbohydrate choices 1

Calories 159

Carbohydrate 13 grams

Protein 20 grams

Fat 3 grams

Saturated Fat <1 gram

Cholesterol 45 milligrams

Sodium 1292 milligrams

Dietary Fiber 2 grams

% calories from

   Protein 50%

   Carbohydrate 33%

   Fat 17%

Food Exchanges: 1 starch, 2 very lean meat

Dijon-Basted Pork Tenderloin

"The greatest dishes are very simple dishes."—Escoffier.
After you experience this pork tenderloin, you will agree!

1 small whole, boneless pork tenderloin
   (approximately 1 1/2 pounds)

Cooking spray

3 tablespoons Dijon mustard

1 1/2 tablespoons Worcestershire sauce

1 teaspoon dried chopped parsley

Preheat oven to 325°. Trim fat from pork tenderloin and place meat on broiler pan coated with cooking spray. In a small bowl, combine mustard, Worcestershire sauce, and parsley. Coat pork with half of mustard mixture. Insert meat thermometer into thickest part of tenderloin. Bake, basting periodically with remaining mustard mixture, for 1 1/2 hours, or until meat thermometer registers 155 degrees and meat is no longer pink.

Makes 6 (4 ounce) servings
Preparation time: 5 minutes
Cooking time: 1 1/2 hours

Nutrient Information (per serving):

Servings per recipe 6

Serving size 4 ounces

Carbohydrate choices 0

Calories 190

Carbohydrate 1 gram

Protein 33 grams

Fat 6 grams

Saturated Fat 2 grams

Cholesterol 78 milligrams

Sodium 291 milligrams

Dietary Fiber <1 gram

% calories from:

Protein 69%

Carbohydrate 2%

Fat 28%

Food Exchanges: 5 very lean meat

Spinach and Ham Bow Tie Pasta

*Bow tie pasta adds interest to this distinct pasta dish.
You will find that by quickly cooking the spinach, some
texture is maintained and mushiness is prevented.*

12 ounces uncooked bow tie pasta

3 tablespoons olive oil

1 teaspoon minced garlic

6 ounces lean ham, sliced in bite-size strips

2 cups sliced fresh mushrooms

10 ounces fresh spinach, coarsely chopped

1/2 teaspoon salt

1/2 teaspoon crushed red pepper flakes

1/2 cup grated fresh Parmesan cheese

Cook pasta according to directions on package, omitting salt.
Heat oil in large nonstick skillet over medium heat. Add garlic
and sauté for 1 minute, taking care not to brown the garlic. Add
ham and heat another 5 minutes. Next add mushrooms and
spinach and continue to cook until spinach wilts, about 5 minutes; stir periodically. Mix in salt and red pepper flakes. Toss
spinach mixture (including liquid) in with drained hot pasta.
Sprinkle with Parmesan cheese.

Makes 5 (2 cup) servings
Preparation time: 25 minutes

Nutrient Information (per serving):

Servings per recipe 5	Cholesterol 40 milligrams
Serving size 2 cups	Sodium 890 milligrams
Carbohydrate choices 1 1/2	Dietary Fiber 2 grams
Calories 270	% calories from:
Carbohydrate 19 grams	Protein 25%
Protein 17 grams	Carbohydrate 28%
Fat 14 grams	Fat 47%
Saturated Fat 3 grams	

Food Exchanges: 1 starch, 1 vegetable, 2 lean meat, 1 fat

Polish Sausage Skillet Supper

A simple and tasty offering that includes meat, vegetables, and potatoes—all in one!

1/2 head green cabbage, thinly sliced

3 medium potatoes, thinly sliced with skin on

1/2 cup chopped onion

1/2 cup diced green onions

1 cup diced carrots

Cooking spray

8 ounces reduced-fat Polish sausage, thinly sliced

2 tablespoons all-purpose flour

16-ounce can fat-free, reduced-sodium chicken broth

1/2 teaspoon salt

1/4 teaspoon black pepper

1/4 teaspoon garlic powder

Place cabbage, potatoes, onions, and carrots in a large nonstick skillet coated with cooking spray. Stir-fry over medium heat for 5 minutes. Add sausage to vegetables. In a separate bowl, whisk together flour, chicken broth, salt, pepper, and garlic powder. Stir into sausage/vegetable mixture and place over high heat. Bring to a boil, then reduce heat and simmer uncovered for 20 minutes, or until potatoes and carrots are tender. Stir periodically to prevent sticking.

Makes 4 (2 cup) servings
Preparation time: 25 minutes
Cooking time: 20 minutes

Nutrient Information (per serving):

Servings per recipe 4	Cholesterol 32 milligrams
Serving size 2 cups	Sodium 876 milligrams
Carbohydrate choices 3 1/2	Dietary Fiber 6 grams
Calories 326	% calories from:
Carbohydrate 53 grams	Protein 18%
Protein 15 grams	Carbohydrate 65%
Fat 6 grams	Fat 17%
Saturated Fat 0	

Food Exchanges: 3 starch, 1 vegetable, 1 lean meat

Western-Style Chicken Pizza

An array of herbs mingles with the tangy taste of barbecue sauce in this imaginative pizza. Smoky grilled chicken, pungent purple onion, and mellow Monterey Jack cheese are toppers that will entice your taste buds!

1 (6 ounce) boneless, skinless chicken breast

1 large Boboli thin pizza crust

3/4 cup barbecue sauce

1/2 small purple onion, sliced and separated into rings

1/2 teaspoon rosemary

1 teaspoon basil

1 teaspoon oregano

1/2 teaspoon tarragon

1 cup shredded reduced-fat Monterey Jack cheese

Grill chicken breast over medium coals about 20 minutes, or until tender and no longer pink inside. Remove from grill and cut in strips. Preheat oven to 375°. Spread pizza crust evenly with barbecue sauce, then top with onion rings and chicken strips. Sprinkle with each of the four herbs and lastly the cheese. Bake for 20 minutes or until cheese is melted and bubbly.

Makes 4 (2 slice) servings
Grilling time (for chicken): 20 minutes
Preparation time: 10 minutes
Baking time: 20 minutes

Nutrient Information (per serving):

Servings per recipe 4	Cholesterol 65 milligrams
Serving size 2 slices	Sodium 1566 milligrams
Carbohydrate choices 4 1/2	Dietary Fiber 0
Calories 529	% calories from:
Carbohydrate 67 grams	Protein 27%
Protein 36 grams	Carbohydrate 51%
Fat 13 grams	Fat 22%
Saturated Fat 4 grams	

Food Exchanges: 4 starch, 3 very lean meat, 2 fat

Chicken & Mushroom Bundles

These artistic creations illustrate that "poultry is for the cook what canvas is for the painter."—Brillat-Savarin

2 Choices

S

4 boneless, skinless chicken breasts, diced into 1/2-inch pieces

1 cup finely chopped onion

2 cups thinly sliced fresh mushrooms

Cooking spray

1/2 cup fat-free sour cream

10 3/4-ounce can reduced-fat cream of chicken soup, undiluted

1/4 teaspoon garlic powder

1/4 teaspoon black pepper

3 8-ounce cans refrigerated reduced-fat crescent rolls

1/2 cup finely shredded part-skim mozzarella cheese

Paprika

Preheat oven to 350°. Place chicken, onion, and mushrooms in a large nonstick skillet coated with cooking spray. Cook over medium heat, stirring constantly, for 5 minutes, or until chicken is tender and no longer pink. Remove chicken mixture from heat. Combine sour cream, soup, garlic powder, and black pepper. Add to chicken mixture; stir well to combine. Set aside.

Unroll crescent rolls and separate into 12 rectangles. In each rectangle, press together perforation to seal. Place 1/8 cup chicken mixture in the center of each rectangle, then sprinkle with 2 teaspoons cheese. Bring corners of rectangles together and twist, pinching the seams to seal and make bundles. Place bundles on a baking sheet coated with cooking spray. Sprinkle each bundle lightly with paprika. Bake for 20 minutes, or until bundles are golden brown.

Makes 12 (1 bundle) servings
Preparation time: 20 minutes
Baking time: 20 minutes

Nutrient Information (per serving):

Servings per recipe 12

Serving size 1 bundle

Carbohydrate choices 2

Calories 330

Carbohydrate 27 grams

Protein 15 grams

Fat 18 grams

Saturated Fat 4 grams

Cholesterol 22 milligrams

Sodium 673 milligrams

Dietary Fiber 1 gram

% calories from:

Protein 18%

Carbohydrate 33%

Fat 49%

Food Exchanges: 2 starch, 1 medium-fat meat, 2 fat

Layered Chicken Salad Olé

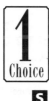

This recipe was inspired by a layered chicken salad that a dear friend of Tami's prepares when Tami drops in for a visit. It rekindles fond memories of fun times. If jalapenos are too fiery for you, decrease the amount or try the milder pickled banana peppers. Serve with crusty, warm bread.

2 whole boneless, skinless chicken breasts

1/4 teaspoon salt

1/2 teaspoon lemon pepper

1 small head iceberg lettuce, chopped (approximately 8 cups)

3/4 cup (3 ounces) shredded reduced-fat Monterey Jack cheese

3/4 cup (3 ounces) shredded reduced-fat cheddar cheese

1/2 cup diced purple onion

1 cup pickled sliced jalapeño peppers

8 ounces reduced-fat ranch-style salad dressing

15 baked tortilla chips, crumbled

Sprinkle chicken breasts with salt and lemon pepper. Grill over medium-hot coals for 24 minutes (12 minutes per side), or until juices run clear and chicken is no longer pink. Remove chicken from grill and cut into bite-size pieces.

In a large salad bowl, place half of chopped lettuce. Layer lettuce with half of the chopped chicken, half of the cheeses, half of the onion, half of the jalapenos, and half of the salad dressing. Repeat layers beginning with lettuce and ending with dressing. If serving immediately, cover top of salad with crumbled tortilla chips. If desired, refrigerate 1 hour before serving to allow flavors to blend, adding chips right before serving.

Makes 6 (2 cup) servings
Preparation time: 30 minutes
Chilling time: 1 hour (optional)

Nutrient Information (per serving):

Servings per recipe 6	Cholesterol 27 milligrams
Serving size 2 cups	Sodium 1071 milligrams
Carbohydrate choices 1	Dietary Fiber 2 grams
Calories 255	% calories from:
Carbohydrate 12 grams	Protein 28%
Protein 18 grams	Carbohydrate 19%
Fat 15 grams	Fat 53%
Saturated Fat 3 grams	

Food Exchanges: 1 starch, 2 lean meat, 1 fat

Chicken and Broccoli Deluxe

A deliciously quick casserole combining the flavors of chicken, stuffing, and broccoli. May be prepared ahead and refrigerated until baking time—increase baking time by 5 minutes.

1 3/4 cups Pepperidge Farm stuffing mix
5 tablespoons reduced-calorie margarine, melted
Cooking spray
10 3/4-ounce can reduced-fat cream of chicken soup
2 cups shredded, cooked chicken breast
1/2 cup skim milk
2 cups frozen chopped broccoli, thawed
1 tablespoon dried instant minced onion
1/8 teaspoon black pepper

Preheat oven to 425°. Place stuffing crumbs and margarine in a bowl and mix until stuffing is moist. Pat all but 3/4 cup of the stuffing mixture into the bottom of a 2-quart casserole dish coated with cooking spray. In a separate bowl, stir together soup, chicken, milk, broccoli, onion, and black pepper. Pour chicken mixture over stuffing layer and top with remaining 3/4 cup stuffing. Bake for 20 minutes, or until bubbly.

Makes 6 (1 cup) servings
Preparation time: 10 minutes
Baking time: 20 minutes

Nutrient Information (per serving):

Servings per recipe 6	Cholesterol 45 milligrams
Serving size 1 cup	Sodium 795 milligrams
Carbohydrate choices 2	Dietary Fiber 3 grams
Calories 257	% calories from:
Carbohydrate 26 grams	Protein 28%
Protein 18 grams	Carbohydrate 40%
Fat 9 grams	Fat 32%
Saturated Fat 2 grams	

Food Exchanges: 1 starch, 2 vegetable, 2 lean meat

Herb-Roasted Chicken

The array of herbs in this recipe scents the kitchen with a wonderful aroma while the chicken is baking.

3 teaspoons canola oil, divided
2 teaspoons crushed garlic
1 1/2 tablespoons crushed dried rosemary
2 teaspoons dried parsley
5 pound roaster chicken
1/4 teaspoon salt
1/4 teaspoon coarse ground pepper

Preheat oven to 350°. In a small bowl, stir together 1 teaspoon oil, garlic, rosemary, and parsley. Rinse the inside and outside of the chicken, then carefully insert your fingers between the skin and flesh, loosening the skin over the entire breast. Using your fingers, spread the herb mixture evenly between the skin and breast.

Brush the remaining 2 teaspoons oil over the entire surface of the chicken. Sprinkle chicken with the salt and pepper. Place chicken in roasting pan, breast side up, and bake uncovered for 1 hour and 45 minutes, or until meat is tender and the juices run clear. If a meat thermometer is used, it should register 185 degrees.

Note: Remove skin before eating to reduce fat content.

Makes 8 (1/8 of chicken) servings
Preparation time: 10 minutes
Baking time: 1 hour and 45 minutes

Nutrient Information (per serving):

(skin included in nutrition analysis)

Servings per recipe 8

Serving size 1/8 of chicken

Carbohydrate choices 0

Calories 292

Carbohydrate 1 gram

Protein 36 grams

Fat 16 grams

Saturated Fat 4 grams

Cholesterol 106 milligrams

Sodium 127 milligrams

Dietary Fiber <1 gram

% calories from:

Protein 49%

Carbohydrate 1%

Fat 49%

Food Exchanges: 5 lean meat

Fiesta Chicken Picante

Dijon mustard and lime juice add zip to this quick and colorful main fare.

8 boneless, skinless chicken breast halves

Cooking spray

3 cups medium picante sauce

2 tablespoons Dijon mustard

1 teaspoon lime juice

4 cups cooked brown rice

1/2 cup (2 ounces) shredded reduced-fat Monterey Jack cheese

1/4 cup chopped green onions

Preheat oven to 400°. Place chicken in a baking dish coated with cooking spray. In a large bowl, mix together picante sauce, mustard, and lime juice. Pour over chicken. Bake for 40 minutes, or until chicken is no longer pink in the center.

To serve, place 1/2 cup rice on each plate and top with a chicken breast half and sauce. Sprinkle with 1 tablespoon cheese and green onions.

Makes 8 (1 chicken breast half, 1/2 cup rice,1 tablespoon cheese) servings
Preparation time: 10 minutes
Baking time: 40 minutes

Nutrient Information (per serving):

Servings per recipe 8

Serving size 1 chicken breast half
   and sauce, 1/2 cup rice,
   1 tablespoon cheese

Carbohydrate choices 2

Calories 307

Carbohydrate 28 grams

Protein 33 grams

Fat 7 grams

Saturated Fat 2 grams

Cholesterol 78 milligrams

Sodium 503 milligrams

Dietary Fiber 2 grams

% calories from:

   Protein 43%

   Carbohydrate 36%

   Fat 21%

Food Exchanges: 2 starch, 4 very lean meat

Turkey Parmesan

Serve with warm crusty French bread and a crisp green salad.

   1/2 cup unseasoned dry bread crumbs

   1/2 teaspoon garlic powder

   1/4 cup grated Parmesan cheese

   1/4 cup liquid egg substitute

   1 pound turkey cutlets

   1/4 teaspoon salt

   Cooking spray

   2 cups fat-free spaghetti sauce

   1 cup (4 ounces) shredded part-skim mozzarella cheese

Preheat oven to 350°. In a pie pan, combine bread crumbs, garlic powder, and parmesan cheese. Pour egg substitute in a bowl.
Sprinkle turkey cutlets with salt. Dip each turkey cutlet in egg
substitute and then coat with bread crumb mixture. Place in a
9" x 13" baking dish coated with cooking spray and top with
spaghetti sauce. Sprinkle with mozzarella cheese. Cover with foil

and bake for 35 minutes, or until bubbly and turkey is no longer pink.

Makes 4 (4 ounce) servings
Preparation time: 15 minutes
Baking time: 35 minutes

Nutrient Information (per serving):

Servings per recipe 4
Serving size 4 ounces
Carbohydrate choices 2 1/2
Calories 468
Carbohydrate 31 grams
Protein 50 grams
Fat 16 grams
Saturated Fat 7 grams

Cholesterol 120 milligrams
Sodium 1155 milligrams
Dietary Fiber 2 grams
% calories from:
  Protein 43%
  Carbohydrate 26%
  Fat 31%

Food Exchanges: 1 starch, 1 vegetable, 1 skim milk, 5 lean meat

Turkey Cutlets in White Wine Sauce

Slice the mushrooms for the sauce quickly and neatly using an egg slicer.

6 (4 ounce) turkey cutlets
1/2 cup all-purpose flour
1 teaspoon crushed dried tarragon
1/8 teaspoon garlic powder
1/4 teaspoon salt
1/4 teaspoon coarse ground pepper
3 tablespoons corn oil
Cooking spray
1/2 cup dry white wine
1 cup water
1/8 teaspoon salt
1/2 cup finely diced onions
2 cups finely sliced mushrooms
2 tablespoons capers

Preheat oven to 375°. Place turkey cutlets between two sheets of waxed paper and flatten to 1/2-inch thickness with a rolling pin or meat mallet. In a large bowl, combine flour, tarragon, garlic powder, salt, and pepper. Place cutlets, one at a time, in flour mixture and turn to coat well. Heat oil in large nonstick skillet coated with cooking spray. Add cutlets and lightly brown on both sides over medium heat. Remove cutlets with a slotted spoon; place in a shallow baking dish coated with cooking spray, then set aside.

Stir remaining flour mixture into drippings in hot skillet (mixture will be thick). Add wine, water, and salt. Increase heat to high and bring to a boil. Reduce heat and cook over medium heat, whisking continuously, until sauce is smooth and thickened. Stir in onions, mushrooms, and capers. Cook until onions are translucent; stirring periodically. Pour sauce over cutlets. Cover with foil and bake for 15 minutes, or until turkey is no longer pink in the center.

Makes 6 (4 ounce) servings
Preparation time: 20 minutes
Baking time: 15 minutes

Nutrient Information (per serving):

Servings per recipe 6
Serving size 4 ounces
Carbohydrate choices 1
Calories 236
Carbohydrate 11 grams
Protein 30 grams
Fat 8 grams
Saturated Fat 1 gram

Cholesterol 70 milligrams
Sodium 309 milligrams
Dietary Fiber <1 gram
% calories from:
　Protein 51%
　Carbohydrate 19%
　Fat 31%

Food Exchanges: 1 starch, 3 lean meat

Turkey for Two in Foil

A simple meal that's baked in a foil packet—no dishes to wash!

Cooking spray
2 (4 ounce) turkey cutlets
1 small onion, sliced and separated into rings
1 medium baking potato, sliced with skin on
1 carrot, peeled and cut in thin sticks
1 stalk celery, cut in thin sticks
1/8 teaspoon dried rosemary
1/8 teaspoon salt
1/2 teaspoon lemon pepper

Preheat oven to 350°. Coat the inside of each of two large pieces heavy-duty aluminum foil with cooking spray. Place a turkey cutlet on each piece of foil. Top each with half of onion, potato, carrot, celery, rosemary, salt, and lemon pepper. Wrap tightly and put in baking pan. Bake for 1 hour and 15 minutes, or until vegetables are tender and turkey is no longer pink.

Makes 2 (1 pouch) servings
Preparation time: 15 minutes
Baking time: 1 hour and 15 minutes

Nutrient Information (per serving):

Servings per recipe 2	Cholesterol 79 milligrams
Serving size 1 pouch	Sodium 258 milligrams
Carbohydrate choices 2 1/2	Dietary Fiber 4 grams
Calories 320	% calories from:
Carbohydrate 34 grams	Protein 46%
Protein 37 grams	Carbohydrate 43%
Fat 4 grams	Fat 11%
Saturated Fat 1 gram	

Food Exchanges: 1 starch, 4 vegetable, 4 very lean meat

Gourmet Peppered-Turkey Bagel Sandwich

A fresh twist on the conventional sandwich. Prepare ahead, then wrap each sandwich in plastic wrap—you're ready for a gourmet picnic!

4 (2 ounce) plain bagels, split

8 tablespoons Dijon-mayonnaise spread

8 ounces peppered turkey, deli sliced

4 leaves green leaf lettuce

4 thin purple onion slices

12 thin cucumber slices

4 tomato slices

16 jalapeno or banana pepper rings

Spread each bagel half with 1 tablespoon Dijon-mayonnaise spread. On bottom halves of bagels, layer 2 ounces turkey, 1 lettuce leaf, 1 onion slice, 3 cucumber slices, 1 tomato slice, 4 pepper rings, and then top halves of bagels. Slice each sandwich in half and serve.

Makes 4 (1 sandwich) servings
Preparation time: 15 minutes

Nutrient Information (per serving):

Servings per recipe 4	Cholesterol 8 milligrams
Serving size 1 sandwich	Sodium 1238 milligrams
Carbohydrate choices 3	Dietary Fiber <1 gram
Calories 328	% calories from:
Carbohydrate 44 grams	Protein 13%
Protein 11 grams	Carbohydrate 54%
Fat 12 grams	Fat 33%
Saturated Fat 2 grams	

Food Exchanges: 3 starch, 1 lean meat, 1 fat

Cranberry Glazed Sirloin Tips over Noodles

Cranberry juice lends a slight sweetness to the glaze over the sirloin tips.

S

2 pounds sirloin tips
Cooking spray
1/3 cup cranberry juice
14 1/2-ounce can beef broth, fat removed
3 tablespoons reduced-sodium soy sauce
1/8 teaspoon ground ginger
1/8 teaspoon garlic powder
1/4 cup cranberry juice
1 tablespoon cornstarch
8 cups cooked no-yolk egg noodles

Cut sirloin into bite-size pieces and place in a large nonstick skillet coated with cooking spray. Brown meat on all sides. Mix in 1/3 cup cranberry juice, beef broth, soy sauce, ginger, and garlic powder. Cover and simmer over low-medium heat for 45 minutes, or until meat is tender; stir periodically throughout cooking. When meat is tender, place remaining cranberry juice in a small bowl. Add cornstarch and stir until dissolved. Pour cornstarch mixture into beef and cook over medium heat, stirring constantly, until sauce is slightly thickened. Serve over noodles.

Makes 8 (4 ounces beef, 1 cup noodles) servings
Preparation time: 20 minutes
Cooking time: 50 minutes

Nutrient Information (per serving):

Servings per recipe 8

Serving size 4 ounces beef, 1 c. noodles

Carbohydrate choices 3 1/2

Calories 433

Carbohydrate 47 grams

Protein 41 grams

Fat 9 grams

Saturated Fat 3 grams

Cholesterol 128 milligrams

Sodium 496 milligrams

Dietary Fiber 3 grams

% calories from:

Protein 38%

Carbohydrate 43%

Fat 18%

Food Exchanges: 3 starch, 4 1/2 very lean meat

Confetti Tamale Casserole

S F

To prepare authentic Mexican tamales, a cornmeal dough is spread in corn husks, then filled with a meat mixture and steamed. Our rendition of this ancient favorite incorporates hash-brown potatoes in place of the cornmeal dough. And, well, an oven works just fine for cooking this creation!

1 pound ground chuck

1/4 cup chopped onion

15 1/2-ounce can red beans, rinsed and drained

15-ounce can shoepeg corn, rinsed and drained

14 1/2-ounce can diced tomatoes

8-ounce can tomato sauce

2 tablespoons chili powder

1 tablespoon cumin

1 tablespoon A-1 steak sauce

1/2 teaspoon Red Hot sauce

1/2 teaspoon salt

3 cups frozen shredded hash-brown potatoes, thawed

2 tablespoons reduced-calorie margarine, melted

Cooking spray

1/2 cup finely grated cheddar cheese

Preheat oven to 350°. In a large skillet combine ground chuck and onion. Cook over medium heat until meat is browned, then drain fat. Add red beans, corn, diced tomatoes, tomato sauce, chili powder, cumin, steak sauce, hot sauce, and salt. Stir to combine and cook over medium heat for 10 minutes.

While meat mixture is cooking, stir together hash-brown potatoes and margarine. Place half the potato mixture in the bottom of a 3-quart casserole dish coated with cooking spray. Add a layer of the meat mixture and top with remaining potatoes. Sprinkle cheese evenly over potatoes and bake for 40 minutes, or until potatoes are lightly browned and casserole is bubbly.

Makes 10 (1 cup) servings
Preparation time: 25 minutes
Baking time: 40 minutes

Nutrient Information (per serving):

Servings per recipe 10	Cholesterol 40 milligrams
Serving size 1 cup	Sodium 471 milligrams
Carbohydrate choices 2	Dietary Fiber 6 grams
Calories 315	% calories from:
Carbohydrate 29 grams	Protein 20%
Protein 16 grams	Carbohydrate 37%
Fat 15 grams	Fat 43%
Saturated Fat 5 grams	

Food Exchanges: 2 starch, 2 medium-fat meat

Stuffed Cabbage Leaves with Tomato Sauce

The practice of wrapping food before placing it into direct heat is nearly as old as cooking itself! Here cabbage leaves provide an edible coating for the savory ground beef and rice filling.

- 1 pound ground chuck
- 1/4 cup chopped onion
- 1 teaspoon Worcestershire sauce
- 1 teaspoon minced garlic
- 1/2 teaspoon dried thyme
- 1 tablespoon dried parsley
- 1/2 teaspoon salt
- 1/8 teaspoon cayenne pepper
- 1 cup cooked brown rice
- 14 cabbage leaves
- Cooking spray
- 8-ounce can tomato sauce
- 1 cup water

Place ground chuck and onion in a large skillet over medium heat. Brown meat, then drain fat. Stir in Worcestershire sauce, garlic, thyme, parsley, salt, cayenne pepper, and rice. Set aside.

Preheat oven to 350°. Place cabbage leaves in a pan of boiling water, remove pan from heat, and allow leaves to sit in water for 5 minutes, or until leaves are wilted (may want to remove tough base of leaves). Drain water off leaves. Place 1/4 cup meat filling on each cabbage leaf. Fold in the two sides of each cabbage leaf and then roll leaf up. Secure with a toothpick. Place cabbage rolls in a 9"x 13" baking dish coated with cooking spray. Pour tomato sauce and water over cabbage rolls and bake for 30 minutes.

Makes 7 (2 cabbage roll) servings
Preparation time: 35 minutes
Baking time: 30 minutes

Nutrient Information (per serving):

Servings per recipe 7

Serving size 2 cabbage rolls

Carbohydrate choices 1

Calories 184

Carbohydrate 12 grams

Protein 16 grams

Fat 8 grams

Saturated Fat 3 grams

Cholesterol 48 milligrams

Sodium 371 milligrams

Dietary Fiber 2 grams

% calories from:

Protein 35%

Carbohydrate 26%

Fat 39%

Food Exchanges: 1 starch, 2 lean meat

Chargrilled Steak and Potatoes on a Stick

S

In addition to this recipe's marinade lending a delicate flavor to the meat, the vinegar in the marinade acts as a tenderizer and the oil a moisturizer. The end result—succulent, juicy steak!

Marinade:

3 tablespoons corn oil

1/3 cup red wine vinegar

1 tablespoon Worcestershire sauce

2 tablespoons reduced-sodium soy sauce

1 tablespoon Dijon mustard

1 teaspoon crushed garlic

1 tablespoon minced dried parsley

1/8 teaspoon coarse ground black pepper

1 pound boneless sirloin steak, cut into 16 1-inch cubes

8 small red-skin potatoes, cut in half

Place marinade ingredients in a bowl and whisk to combine. Put steak cubes in a large zip-top plastic bag and pour half of marinade over steak. Close bag securely and refrigerate overnight, or 8 hours, shaking bag gently twice during marinating. Reserve remaining marinade in covered container in refrigerator.

When ready to assemble skewers, place potatoes in a saucepan then cover with water and lid. Bring to a boil over high heat. Reduce heat and simmer for 10 minutes, or until tender but not mushy. Drain, place in bowl, and toss with reserved marinade. Thread each of four skewers with 4 steak cubes and 4 potato halves, beginning with steak and ending with potato. Grill skewers over hot coals for 5 minutes per side, basting with remaining marinade from potatoes. Do not use remaining marinade from meat.

Makes 4 (1 skewer) servings
Preparation time: 20 minutes
Marinating time: 8 hours
Cooking time: 10 minutes

Nutrient Information (per serving):

Servings per recipe 4

Serving size 1 skewer

Carbohydrate choices 3

Calories 564

Carbohydrate 43 grams

Protein 35 grams

Fat 28 grams

Saturated Fat 8 grams

Cholesterol 102 milligrams

Sodium 475 milligrams

Dietary Fiber 3 grams

% calories from:

Protein 25%

Carbohydrate 30%

Fat 45%

Food Exchanges: 3 starch, 5 lean meat, 1 fat

Pizza Meat Loaf

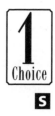

The merging of two of America's favorites—pizza and meat loaf! Time-saving tip: Combine raw meat loaf ingredients, place in loaf pan, and store in refrigerator until baking time.

1 1/2 pounds ground chuck

1/2 cup dry unseasoned bread crumbs

1/2 cup liquid egg substitute

1 tablespoon instant chopped onion

1/4 teaspoon black pepper

1/2 teaspoon salt

1/2 teaspoon garlic salt

1/2 teaspoon crushed dried oregano

Cooking spray

14-ounce jar pizza sauce

7-ounce can sliced mushrooms, drained

1/2 cup finely shredded part-skim mozzarella cheese

Preheat oven to 375°. In large mixing bowl, knead together first 8 ingredients. Press into a large loaf pan coated with cooking spray. Bake for 45 minutes. Remove from oven and drain off drippings. Top with pizza sauce, followed by mushrooms, then cheese. Return to oven and bake an additional 25 minutes, or until sauce is bubbly and cheese is melted. Cut into 9 slices and serve.

Makes 9 (1-inch slice) servings
Preparation time: 5 minutes
Baking time: 1 hour and 10 minutes

Nutrient Information (per serving):

Servings per recipe 9	Cholesterol 60 milligrams
Serving size 1 (1 inch) slice	Sodium 518 milligrams
Carbohydrate choices 1	Dietary Fiber 2 grams
Calories 274	% calories from:
Carbohydrate 9 grams	Protein 28%
Protein 19 grams	Carbohydrate 13%
Fat 18 grams	Fat 59%
Saturated Fat 7 grams	

Food Exchanges: 1/2 starch, 2 medium-fat meat, 1 fat

Peppery Beef Roast with Gravy

"The feeling of friendship is like that of being comfortably filled with roast beef."—Samuel Johnson

0
Choices

1 (4 pound) rump roast, fat trimmed
1 teaspoon salt
1/2 teaspoon garlic powder
2 teaspoons coarse ground black pepper
1 tablespoon instant chopped onion
Cooking spray

Gravy:

2 tablespoons reduced-calorie stick margarine
1/3 cup all-purpose flour
1/2 cup cold water
1 cup reduced-sodium, fat-free beef bouillon
1/3 cup dry red wine
1/8 teaspoon black pepper

Preheat oven to 325°. Rub roast with salt, garlic powder, and black pepper. Sprinkle with onion. Place roast in a shallow roasting pan coated with cooking spray and insert meat thermometer into roast. Bake for 2 hours, or until meat is tender and meat thermometer registers 160 to 170 degrees. Remove roast from oven and keep warm.

To make gravy, melt margarine in a saucepan over medium heat. In a small bowl, combine flour and cold water using a wire whisk to remove lumps. Pour flour mixture through a sieve into melted margarine; whisk together. Add beef bouillon and wine; whisk to remove lumps. Cook over medium heat while stirring constantly. Cook about 5 minutes, or until slightly thickened. Slice roast and serve with warm gravy.

Makes 13 (5 ounce) servings
Preparation time: 20 minutes
Baking time: 2 hours

Nutrient Information (per serving):

Servings per recipe 13 servings

Serving size 5 ounces

Carbohydrate choices 0

Calories 295

Carbohydrate 3 grams

Protein 42 grams

Fat 12 grams

Saturated Fat 4 grams

Cholesterol 103 milligrams

Sodium 314 milligrams

Dietary Fiber <1 gram

% calories from:

Protein 57%

Carbohydrate 4%

Fat 37%

Alcohol: 2%

Food Exchanges: 6 lean meat

Chili Italiano

*"Next to jazz music, there is nothing that lifts the spirit
and strengthens the soul more than a good bowl of chili."*
—Harry James

1 pound ground chuck

1 cup chopped onion (approximately 1/2 of a large onion)

27.5-ounce jar light mushroom pasta sauce

1/2 teaspoon crushed dried oregano

1/2 teaspoon salt

3 cups very low sodium beef bouillon

15-1/2 ounce can red beans, rinsed and drained

3 cups cooked penne pasta (approximately 6 ounces uncooked)

Place meat and onion in a large nonstick skillet and brown over medium heat. Crumble meat as it cooks. Drain fat and place meat in a stockpot. Add pasta sauce, oregano, salt, bouillon, and red beans. Stir to combine and cook uncovered over medium heat for 20 minutes. Add cooked pasta and serve.

Makes 5 1/2 (2 cup) servings
Preparation time: 20 minutes
Cooking time: 20 minutes

Nutrient Information (per serving):

Servings per recipe 5 1/2

Serving size 2 cups

Carbohydrate choices 3

Calories 433

Carbohydrate 45 grams

Protein 25 grams

Fat 17 grams

Saturated Fat 6 grams

Cholesterol 57 milligrams

Sodium 979 milligrams

Dietary Fiber 9 grams

% calories from:

    Protein 23%

    Carbohydrate 42%

    Fat 35%

Food Exchanges: 2 starch, 2 1/2 lean meat, 1 fat

Sensational Stuffed Flounder

*Seasoned, moist stuffing nicely complements
this tender, flaky fish.*

$\frac{1}{2}$ Choice

2/3 cup water

1 tablespoon reduced-calorie margarine

1 cup dry stuffing mix

Cooking spray

2 (8 ounce) flounder fillets

1/8 teaspoon coarse ground black pepper

2 teaspoons lemon juice

2 tablespoons reduced-calorie margarine, melted

Preheat oven to 400°. Place water and 1 tablespoon margarine in a saucepan; bring to a boil. Stir in stuffing mix. Cover, and remove from heat. Allow to stand 5 minutes, then fluff with a fork.

Place a baking rack coated with cooking spray in a baking dish. Lay flounder on rack and sprinkle with pepper and lemon juice. Spoon half of stuffing on top of each fillet. Drizzle fish with the 2 tablespoons melted margarine. Bake for 15 minutes, or until fish flakes easily with a fork.

Makes 4 (4 ounces flounder, 1/4 cup stuffing) servings
Preparation time: 15 minutes
Baking time: 15 minutes

Nutrient Information (per serving):

Servings per recipe 4	Saturated Fat 1 gram
Serving size 4 ounces flounder,	Cholesterol 72 milligrams
1/4 cup stuffing	Sodium 367 milligrams
Carbohydrate choices 1/2	Dietary Fiber 0
Calories 194	% calories from:
Carbohydrate 8 grams	Protein 56%
Protein 27 grams	Carbohydrate 16%
Fat 6 grams	Fat 28%

Food Exchanges: 1/2 starch, 3 lean meat

Marjoram Baked Halibut with Parmesan Crumb Topping

1/2 Choice

The marjoram in this recipe lends a spicy, slightly sweet flavor to the Parmesan cheese topping.

2 pounds halibut

Cooking spray

2 tablespoons lemon juice

1/4 teaspoon salt

1/2 teaspoon black pepper

1/2 cup dry unseasoned bread crumbs

2 teaspoons minced garlic

3 tablespoons canola oil

3 tablespoons grated Parmesan cheese

1/4 teaspoon crushed dried marjoram

Preheat oven to 450°. Place halibut in a baking dish coated with cooking spray. Sprinkle with lemon juice, salt, and pepper, then set aside. In a bowl, mix together bread crumbs, garlic, oil, Parmesan cheese, and marjoram to make a thick paste. Pat

Parmesan mixture onto fish. Bake for 15 minutes, or until fish flakes easily with a fork.

Makes 8 (4 ounce) servings
Preparation time: 8 minutes
Baking time: 15 minutes

Nutrient Information (per serving):

Servings per recipe 8

Serving size 4 ounce

Carbohydrate choices 1/2

Calories 242

Carbohydrate 6 grams

Protein 32 grams

Fat 10 grams

Saturated Fat 1 gram

Cholesterol 49 milligrams

Sodium 248 milligrams

Dietary Fiber <1 gram

% calories from:

Protein 53%

Carbohydrate 10%

Fat 37%

Food Exchanges: 1/2 starch, 4 very lean meat, 1 fat

Aloha Orange Roughy

"Fish should smell like the tide. Once they smell like fish, it's too late."—Oscar Gizelt
These are wise words to keep in mind when purchasing fish. A fresh fish should have reddish gills, eyes that are bulging, firm flesh, scales that are shiny and adhere firmly to the skin, and no strong odor.

16 ounce orange roughy fillet

1/4 cup pineapple juice

2 tablespoons steak sauce

1/4 teaspoon salt

1/8 teaspoon pepper

Cooking spray

2 tablespoons slivered almonds, toasted

Place fish in a baking dish. In a small bowl, combine pineapple juice, steak sauce, salt, and pepper. Pour over fish and marinate in refrigerator for 30 minutes, turning once. Remove fish from marinade and place on broiler pan coated with cooking spray. Broil for 2 minutes, brush with marinade, and broil an additional 2 minutes. Carefully turn fish over and brush with marinade. Broil an additional 5 minutes, or until fish flakes easily with a fork. Sprinkle cooked fish with slivered almonds.

Makes 4 (4 ounce) servings
Preparation time: 5 minutes
Marinating time: 30 minutes
Cooking time: 9 minutes

Nutrient Information (per serving):

Servings per recipe 4	Cholesterol 29 milligrams
Serving size 4 ounce	Sodium 299 milligrams
Carbohydrate choices 0	Dietary Fiber <1 gram
Calories 131	% calories from:
Carbohydrate 4 grams	Protein 67%
Protein 22 grams	Carbohydrate 12%
Fat 3 grams	Fat 21%
Saturated Fat <1 gram	

Food Exchanges: 1/2 fruit, 3 very lean meat

Diablo Shrimp

A must for those who love fiery flavors! Also can be tossed with steaming linguini for pasta lovers.

0
Choices

S

3 tablespoons reduced-calorie margarine
Cooking spray
1 teaspoon chili powder
1/2 teaspoon ground cumin
1/8 teaspoon cayenne pepper
1 teaspoon lemon pepper
1/4 teaspoon dried dillweed
1 pound fresh shrimp, peeled

Melt margarine over medium heat in a large nonstick skillet coated with cooking spray. Stir chili powder, cumin, cayenne pepper, lemon pepper, and dillweed into margarine. Add shrimp and continue cooking over medium heat, stirring constantly. Cook for 4 minutes, or until shrimp curl slightly and are tender.

Makes 4 servings
Preparation time: 5 minutes
Cooking time: 4 minutes

Nutrient Information (per serving):

Servings per recipe 4
Serving size 1/4 recipe
Carbohydrate choices 0
Calories 132
Carbohydrate 1 gram
Protein 23 grams
Fat 4 grams
Saturated Fat 1 gram

Cholesterol 173 milligrams
Sodium 884 milligrams
Dietary Fiber <1 gram
% calories from:
  Protein 70%
  Carbohydrate 3%
  Fat 27%

Food Exchanges: 3 very lean meat

Sautéed Sea Scallops with Angel Hair Pasta

1½ Choices

S

A hint of sage complements the sweet-tasting scallops in this beautiful pasta.

- 1 tablespoon + 1 teaspoon corn oil
- 8 Roma tomatoes, chopped with seeds removed
- 1/2 teaspoon salt
- 1/8 teaspoon cayenne pepper
- 1 teaspoon crushed garlic
- 1/4 teaspoon coarse ground black pepper
- 1/4 teaspoon dried rubbed sage
- Cooking spray
- 2 tablespoons reduced-calorie margarine
- 40 sea scallops (approximately 1/2 pound), drained
- 1/2 pound angel hair pasta, cooked according to package directions (omit salt)
- 4 teaspoons grated fat-free Parmesan cheese

Place oil in a nonstick skillet over medium heat. Add tomatoes, salt, and cayenne pepper; cook for 3 minutes, stirring periodically. Add garlic, black pepper, and sage and cook for 2 additional minutes, stirring constantly. Set aside.

In another nonstick skillet coated with cooking spray, melt margarine. Add scallops, and sauté over medium heat until they are no longer translucent. Place a fourth of the pasta on each plate and top with 10 scallops. Spoon tomato sauce over the scallops, and top with 1 teaspoon Parmesan cheese.

Makes 4 servings
Preparation time: 20 minutes

Nutrient Information (per serving):

Servings per recipe 4	Cholesterol 30 milligrams
Serving size 1/4 recipe	Sodium 502 milligrams
Carbohydrate choices 1 1/2	Dietary Fiber 1 gram
Calories 245	% calories from:
Carbohydrate 23 grams	Protein 29%
Protein 18 grams	Carbohydrate 38%
Fat 9 grams	Fat 33%
Saturated Fat 1 gram	

Food Exchanges: 1 starch, 2 vegetable, 2 lean meat

Under the Sea Sandwich

*A great substitute for a burger if you are limiting red meat.
Top with your favorite burger fixings.*

S

> 2 9-ounce cans white tuna in spring water,
>   drained and flaked
> 1 cup fresh bread crumbs
> 1/2 cup liquid egg substitute
> 1/4 cup finely diced celery
> 1/4 cup finely diced onion
> 1/4 cup skim milk
> 1 teaspoon chopped dried parsley
> 1/2 teaspoon garlic salt
> 1/8 teaspoon cayenne pepper
> 1/2 cup fine, dry seasoned bread crumbs
> Butter-flavored cooking spray
> 7 sesame seed hamburger buns

Preheat oven to 350°. In a large bowl, combine tuna, fresh bread
crumbs, egg substitute, celery, onion, milk, parsley, garlic salt, and
pepper; mix well. Place dry bread crumbs in a separate shallow
bowl. Shape tuna mixture into 7 patties (uncooked patties will
break apart easily). Cover patties with the dry bread crumbs by
laying patties in bread crumbs and gently turning once to coat.
Place tuna patties on a baking sheet coated with cooking spray.

Lightly spray tops of patties with cooking spray. Bake for 30 minutes, or until lightly browned. Serve on hamburger buns.

Makes 7 (1 patty) servings
Preparation time: 10 minutes
Baking time: 30 minutes

Nutrient Information (per serving):

Servings per recipe 7

Serving size 1 patty

Carbohydrate choices 2 1/2

Calories 302

Carbohydrate 34 grams

Protein 28 grams

Fat 6 grams

Saturated Fat <1 gram

Cholesterol 31 milligrams

Sodium 616 milligrams

Dietary Fiber 1 gram

% calories from:

Protein 37%

Carbohydrate 45%

Fat 18%

Food Exchanges: 2 starch, 3 lean meat

Tuna and Shells Toss

A light and refreshing main dish.

7 ounces uncooked small pasta shells

3 cups bite-size broccoli florets

12-ounce can tuna packed in spring water, drained and flaked

4 Roma tomatoes, seeded and diced

1/3 cup diced purple onion

3 ounces provolone cheese, finely shredded

2 tablespoons corn oil

1/4 cup + 2 tablespoons red wine vinegar

1/2 teaspoon crushed dried oregano

1/2 teaspoon dried basil

1/4 teaspoon coarse ground black pepper

1/4 teaspoon salt

Bring 2 quarts water to boil over high heat. Reduce heat to medium-high and add pasta shells. Cook 6 minutes, add broccoli, and continue to cook an additional 2 minutes, or until pasta is tender.

Drain and place in large serving bowl. Add tuna, tomatoes, onion, and cheese. Toss to combine. In a small jar, combine oil, vinegar, oregano, basil, pepper, and salt. Cover tightly with lid and shake well. Drizzle over tuna mixture and toss to coat. Chill 1 hour.

Makes 8 (1 cup) servings
Preparation time: 15 minutes
Cooking time: 8 minutes
Chilling time: 1 hour

Nutrient Information (per serving):

Servings per recipe 8	Cholesterol 7 milligrams
Serving size 1 cup	Sodium 332 milligrams
Carbohydrate choices 2	Dietary Fiber 2 grams
Calories 243	% calories from:
Carbohydrate 25 grams	Protein 33%
Protein 20 grams	Carbohydrate 41%
Fat 7 grams	Fat 26%
Saturated Fat 2 grams	

Food Exchanges: 1 1/2 starch, 2 lean meat

Cantina Pasta Salad

Lasagna noodles add a unique twist to this colorful pasta salad.

2 Choices

S **F**

- 3/4 cup reduced-fat sour cream
- 4-ounce can chopped green chilies
- 1/2 teaspoon chili powder
- 1 teaspoon ground cumin
- 9 lasagna noodles, cooked and drained
- 1 pound 13-ounce can pinto beans, rinsed and drained
- 11-ounce can Mexican-style corn, drained
- 4 cups shredded iceberg lettuce
- 16-ounce jar mild salsa
- 3/4 cup finely shredded Monterey Jack cheese
- 1/4 cup reduced-fat sour cream

In a small bowl, combine 3/4 cup sour cream, green chilies, chili powder, and cumin. Set aside.

Place 3 lasagna noodles in the bottom of a 9" x 13" dish. Top with one-third of beans, one-third of corn, and one-third of lettuce. Dollop with one-half of salsa. Sprinkle with one-third of cheese. Repeat layers, substituting sour cream mixture for salsa. Repeat layers again with remaining noodles, beans, corn, lettuce, salsa, and cheese. With remaining 1/4 cup sour cream, put 1 dollop on each serving of salad. Cover and chill 1 hour to allow flavors to blend.

Makes 12 (1 square) servings
Preparation time: 20 minutes
Chilling time: 1 hour

Nutrient Information (per serving):

Servings per recipe 12

Serving size 1 square

Carbohydrate choices 2

Calories 209

Carbohydrate 25 grams

Protein 16 grams

Fat 5 grams

Saturated Fat 3 grams

Cholesterol 14 milligrams

Sodium 1585 milligrams

Dietary Fiber 6 grams

% calories from:

Protein 31%

Carbohydrate 48%

Fat 22%

Food Exchanges: 1 1/2 starch, 2 lean meat

Veggie Jambalaya

Traditional jambalaya is a main dish mixture of rice, beef, pork, chicken, shrimp, crayfish, Cajun seasonings, and any other number of ingredients. So, who would think it possible to have great-tasting jambalaya without all the meat and fat? Here it is! Black-eyed peas replace meat as the protein source—they add extra fiber, too.

2 tablespoons corn oil

Cooking spray

1 cup coarsely diced onion

2 teaspoons minced garlic

3/4 cup coarsely diced celery

1/2 cup diced carrots

1 teaspoon dried thyme

2 teaspoons paprika

1/2 teaspoon salt

1/8 teaspoon cayenne pepper

1 bay leaf

1 red pepper, seeded and cut into strips

15-ounce can black-eyed peas, undrained

14 1/2-ounce can diced tomatoes, undrained

2 14 1/2-ounce cans reduced-sodium, fat-free chicken broth

2 medium-size zucchini, coarsely diced

1 1/2 cups uncooked long-grain white rice

2 tablespoons chopped parsley

Heat oil in a large nonstick skillet coated with cooking spray. Add onion and cook over low heat until translucent, about 8 minutes. Add garlic, celery, and carrots and cook 1 minute longer, stirring periodically. Mix in the next 5 ingredients, then add the red pepper, black-eyed peas, tomatoes, and broth. Bring to a boil. Reduce heat to medium and cook, partially covered, for 10 minutes. Next, add the zucchini and bring to a boil once again. Stir in the rice, cover, reduce heat to low, and cook for 20 minutes. Remove bay leaf and toss in parsley. Serve immediately.

Makes 6 (2 cup) servings
Preparation time: 20 minutes
Cooking time: 50 minutes

Nutrient Information (per serving):

Servings per recipe 6	Cholesterol 2 milligrams
Serving size 2 cups	Sodium 292 milligrams
Carbohydrate choices 4	Dietary Fiber 7 grams
Calories 323	% calories from:
Carbohydrate 55 grams	Protein 12%
Protein 10 grams	Carbohydrate 68%
Fat 7 grams	Fat 20%
Saturated Fat 1 gram	

Food Exchanges: 3 starch, 2 vegetable, 1 fat

Barbecue Vegetable Pita Pockets

A fantastic meatless meal!

  1 tablespoon corn oil
  1 large onion, thinly sliced and separated into rings
  1 green pepper, sliced into thin strips
  3 cups sliced fresh mushrooms (approximately 8 ounces)
  1 zucchini, sliced into thin 3-inch strips
  1/2 cup barbecue sauce
  8 pita pockets (halves, not rounds), warmed
  1 cup shredded reduced-fat Monterey Jack cheese

Heat corn oil in a large nonstick skillet over medium heat. Add onion and pepper and cook for 3 minutes; stir periodically during cooking. Add mushrooms and zucchini, then cook for an additional 3 minutes. Stir in barbecue sauce and continue to cook over low heat for 5 minutes, again, stirring periodically. Distribute vegetable mixture evenly between pita pockets (approximately 1/2 cup vegetables per pocket) and sprinkle each pocket with 2 tablespoons cheese.

Makes 8 (1 filled pita pocket) servings
Preparation time: 20 minutes

Nutrient Information (per serving):

Servings per recipe 8	Cholesterol 10 milligrams
Serving size 1 filled pita pocket	Sodium 351 milligrams
Carbohydrate choices 1 1/2	Dietary Fiber 5 grams
Calories 173	% calories from:
Carbohydrate 22 grams	Protein 23%
Protein 10 grams	Carbohydrate 51%
Fat 5 grams	Fat 26%
Saturated Fat 2 grams	

Food Exchanges: 1 1/2 starch, 1 very lean meat

Mediterranean Eggplant Bake

This recipe includes healthy ingredients from traditional Mediterranean fare—eggplant, olive oil, and feta cheese.

1 small eggplant (about 1 pound), peeled and sliced in 1/2-inch-thick slices
Cooking spray
1/8 teaspoon black pepper
1/2 teaspoon salt
2 medium tomatoes, thickly sliced
1 medium onion, thinly sliced and separated into rings
1 tablespoon olive oil
1 teaspoon crushed garlic
1 teaspoon crushed dried oregano
2 ounces shredded part-skim mozzarella cheese
2 ounces (1/4 cup) crumbled feta cheese
Paprika

Heat oven broiler. Place eggplant slices on a baking pan coated with cooking spray. Sprinkle with pepper and salt. Broil 5 inches from heat source (with oven door partially open) for 6 minutes, or until lightly browned. Remove from oven and decrease oven temperature to 375°.

Coat a 10-inch pie plate with cooking spray and line with the eggplant slices, browned-side down. Overlap slices in a circular pattern. Alternate slices of tomato and onion over the eggplant. In a small cup, combine oil and garlic. Drizzle over vegetables. Sprinkle with oregano. Bake 25 minutes. Sprinkle with mozzarella cheese, feta cheese, and paprika. Bake an additional 10 minutes, or until cheese is melted. Cut into 6 wedges.

Makes 6 (1 wedge) servings
Preparation time: 20 minutes
Baking time: 41 minutes

Nutrient Information (per serving):

Servings per recipe 6	Cholesterol 14 milligrams
Serving size 1 wedge	Sodium 350 milligrams
Carbohydrate choices 1	Dietary Fiber 3 grams
Calories 114	% calories from:
Carbohydrate 10 grams	Protein 18%
Protein 5 grams	Carbohydrate 35%
Fat 6 grams	Fat 47%
Saturated Fat 3 grams	

Food Exchanges: 2 vegetable, 1 fat

Sicilian Spinach-Potato Bake

A twist on lasagna for vegetable lovers. Thinly-sliced red potatoes take the place of lasagna noodles.

10-ounce package frozen spinach, thawed and well drained

1 cup grated carrot

1/2 cup finely chopped onion

15-ounce carton nonfat ricotta cheese

1 teaspoon crushed dried oregano

1/2 teaspoon coarse ground black pepper

1/4 teaspoon salt

Cooking spray

1 1/2 pounds large red potatoes, thinly sliced with skin on

1 cup finely shredded part-skim mozzarella cheese

1/2 cup freshly grated Romano cheese

Paprika

Preheat oven to 375°. In a large bowl, combine spinach, carrot, onion, ricotta cheese, oregano, pepper, and salt. Set aside.

Coat a 9"x 9" baking dish with cooking spray. Place one-third of potato slices in bottom of baking dish. Top with half of spinach mixture, then half of mozzarella cheese. Repeat layers. Top with remaining potato slices and sprinkle with Romano cheese, then paprika. Cover with foil and bake for 30 minutes. Uncover and bake an additional 40 minutes, or until potato is golden and tender when pierced with a fork. To allow for easier serving, let stand for 10 minutes after removed from oven. Cut into six equal portions.

Makes 6 servings
Preparation time: 15 minutes
Baking time: 70 minutes
Standing time: 10 minutes

Nutrient Information (per serving):

Servings per recipe 6	Cholesterol 27 milligrams
Serving size 1/6 recipe	Sodium 494 milligrams
Carbohydrate choices 2 1/2	Dietary Fiber 5 grams
Calories 294	% calories from:
Carbohydrate 38 grams	Protein 30%
Protein 22 grams	Carbohydrate 52%
Fat 6 grams	Fat 18%
Saturated Fat 4 grams	

Food Exchanges: 2 starch, 1 vegetable, 2 lean meat

Easy Vegetable Quiche

Marvelous for brunch or as a light dinner entree. Great accompaniments are Strawberry Spinach Salad with Toasted Almonds (page 70) and Pumpkin Spice Muffins (page 52).

1 1/2 cups frozen chopped broccoli, thawed
1/4 cup grated carrot
1/4 cup chopped red bell pepper
1 cup sliced fresh mushrooms
1/2 cup chopped onion
1/3 cup shredded reduced-fat cheddar cheese
Cooking spray
1 1/2 cups skim milk
3/4 cup baking mix
3/4 cup liquid egg substitute
1/4 teaspoon black pepper
1/2 teaspoon salt

Preheat oven to 400°. In a medium bowl, combine broccoli, carrot, red pepper, mushrooms, onion, and cheese. Place in a quiche dish coated with cooking spray. In a separate bowl, combine milk, baking mix, egg substitute, black pepper, and salt. Beat with an electric mixer until smooth. Pour into quiche dish over vegetables. Bake for 25 to 30 minutes, or until knife inserted 2 inches from edge comes out clean. Let stand 5 minutes before cutting and serving.

Makes 6 (1 slice) servings
Preparation time: 15 minutes
Baking time: 30 minutes

Nutrient Information (per serving):

Servings per recipe 6

Serving size 1/6 of recipe

Carbohydrate choices 1 1/2

Calories 153

Carbohydrate 16 grams

Protein 11 grams

Fat 5 grams

Saturated Fat 1 gram

Cholesterol 6 milligrams

Sodium 505 milligrams

Dietary Fiber 2 grams

% calories from:

   Protein 29%

   Carbohydrate 42%

   Fat 29%

Food Exchanges: 1 starch, 1 medium-fat meat

Top of the Morning Casserole

Makes breakfast a snap since all the preparation is done the night before!

    2 tablespoons reduced-calorie margarine

    1 medium onion, diced

    1/2 pound fresh asparagus, cut into 1-inch pieces

    1 medium red pepper, diced

    2 cups thinly sliced fresh mushrooms

    Cooking spray

    1 loaf French bread, cubed (about 8 cups)

    3 ounces Canadian bacon, diced

    2 cups shredded reduced-fat cheddar cheese

    2 cups liquid egg substitute

    2 1/2 cups skim milk

    1/2 teaspoon salt

    1/2 teaspoon black pepper

In a medium nonstick skillet, melt margarine and then sauté onion, asparagus, red pepper, and mushrooms in margarine for 4 minutes. Coat a 9"x 13" baking dish with cooking spray and layer bread cubes, Canadian bacon, 1 cup cheese, and sautéed vegetables in baking dish. In a medium bowl, whisk together egg substitute, milk, salt, and pepper. Pour mixture evenly over layers and sprinkle with remaining cheese. Cover with plastic wrap and refrigerate 8 hours, or overnight.

Preheat oven to 350°. Bake uncovered for 45 minutes, or until light golden. Cut into 15 squares before serving.

Makes 15 (1 square) servings
Preparation time: 20 minutes
Chilling time: 8 hours
Baking time: 45 minutes

Nutrient Information (per serving):

Servings per recipe 15	Cholesterol 4 milligrams
Serving size 1 square	Sodium 448 milligrams
Carbohydrate choices 1	Dietary Fiber 1 gram
Calories 135	% calories from:
Carbohydrate 14 grams	Protein 39%
Protein 13 grams	Carbohydrate 41%
Fat 3 grams	Fat 20%
Saturated Fat <1 gram	

Food Exchanges: 1/2 starch, 1 vegetable, 1 lean meat

Spicy Black Bean and Rice Soup

4 Choices

S F

"Soup is cuisine's kindest course."—Kitchen Graffiti

3 15-ounce cans black beans, rinsed and drained

3 cups reduced-sodium chicken bouillon

3 tablespoons red wine vinegar

1 teaspoon salt

1 cup uncooked instant brown rice

2 tablespoons olive oil

1 large onion, finely chopped

1 tablespoon minced garlic

1 1/2 teaspoons ground cumin

1/4 teaspoon cayenne pepper

1 teaspoon crushed dried oregano

6 tablespoons reduced-fat sour cream

3 green onions, diced

Place 2 cups beans and 1/2 cup chicken bouillon in food processor and process until smooth. Place bean purée along with remaining beans and chicken bouillon, vinegar, salt, and rice in large stockpot and set aside.

Heat olive oil in a large nonstick skillet. Add onion, garlic, cumin, cayenne pepper, and oregano, and cook over medium heat for 5 minutes, or until onion is translucent; stir frequently. Add onion mixture to bean mixture and simmer uncovered over low-medium heat for 20 minutes to allow flavors to blend; stir periodically. Soup will thicken with cooking; may thin with water if desired. Top each bowl of soup with 1 tablespoon sour cream and a sprinkle of diced green onions.

Makes 6 (1 cup) servings
Preparation time: 15 minutes
Cooking time: 20 minutes

Nutrient Information (per serving):

Servings per recipe 6

Serving size 1 cup

Carbohydrate choices 4

Calories 364

Carbohydrate 59 grams

Protein 14 grams

Fat 8 grams

Saturated Fat 1 grams

Cholesterol 7 milligrams

Sodium 1325 milligrams

Dietary Fiber 11 grams

% calories from:

Protein 15%

Carbohydrate 65%

Fat 20%

Food Exchanges: 4 starch, 1 fat

Navy Bean and Ham Soup

Serve with a thick slice of warm, crusty bread.

16 ounces dried navy beans, rinsed

8 cups water

8 ounces lean ham, finely diced

2 stalks celery, finely diced

1 small onion, finely diced

1 carrot, peeled and finely diced

6 cups water

3/4 teaspoon coarse ground black pepper

1 1/4 teaspoons salt

1/4 teaspoon garlic powder

Combine navy beans, 8 cups water, ham, celery, onion, and carrot in a stockpot and bring to a boil. Reduce heat to medium and cook for 1 1/2 hours, stirring periodically to prevent sticking. Add remaining 6 cups of water as beans absorb water. Add pepper, salt, and garlic powder to soup. Reduce heat to low-medium and continue cooking an additional 30 minutes. During this last half hour of cooking, some navy beans may be mashed with the back of a spoon for a thicker soup.

Makes 9 (1 cup) servings
Preparation time: 20 minutes
Cooking time: 2 hours

Nutrient Information (per serving):

Servings per recipe 9

Serving size 1 cup

Carbohydrate choices 2

Calories 206

Carbohydrate 30 grams

Protein 17 grams

Fat 2 grams

Saturated Fat <1 gram

Cholesterol 14 milligrams

Sodium 686 milligrams

Dietary Fiber 12 grams

% calories from:

Protein 33%

Carbohydrate 58%

Fat 9%

Food Exchanges: 2 starch, 1 1/2 very lean meat

Texas Tortilla Soup

The ingredient list is long, but don't let that discourage you! This tasty soup can be thrown together in just a few moments and you'll only dirty one pan!

2 tablespoons corn oil

I small onion, diced

4 1/2-ounce can chopped green chilies

2 teaspoons minced garlic

14 1/2-ounce can diced tomatoes

2 14 1/2-ounce cans fat-free, reduced-sodium chicken broth

I 1/2 cups water

I cup tomato juice

I teaspoon lemon juice

I teaspoon ground cumin

1/2 teaspoon chili powder

1/4 teaspoon pepper

2 teaspoons Worcestershire sauce

3 6-inch corn tortillas, cut into 1/2-inch strips

3/4 cup + 2 tablespoons shredded reduced-fat cheddar cheese

Heat oil in a large pot. Add onion, chilies, and garlic. Cook over medium heat for 5 minutes, or until onion is soft; stir frequently. Add tomatoes, broth, water, tomato juice, lemon juice, cumin, chili powder, pepper, and Worcestershire sauce to onion mixture. Place over high heat and bring to a boil. Reduce heat to medium and simmer, covered, for 45 minutes. Add tortilla strips and simmer uncovered 10 minutes longer. Top each bowl of soup with 2 tablespoons shredded cheese.

Makes 7 (I cup) servings
Preparation time: 10 minutes
Cooking time: 55 minutes

Nutrient Information (per serving):

Servings per recipe 7

Serving size 1 cup

Carbohydrate choices 1

Calories 125

Carbohydrate 12 grams

Protein 8 grams

Fat 5 grams

Saturated Fat <1 gram

Cholesterol 2 milligrams

Sodium 611 milligrams

Dietary Fiber 2 grams

% calories from:

Protein 26%

Carbohydrate 41%

Fat 33%

Food Exchanges: 1 starch, 1 lean meat

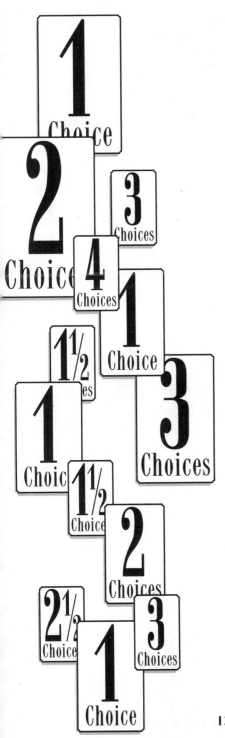

Side Dishes

Rosemary Red-Skin Potatoes and Sugar Snap Peas

$1\frac{1}{2}$ Choices

Rosemary lends a pungent, somewhat minty flavor to this vegetable medley. If you replace dried rosemary with fresh rosemary, use twice the amount.

- 2 pounds small red-skin potatoes
- 4 tablespoons reduced-calorie margarine
- I teaspoon salt
- 1/2 teaspoon coarse ground black pepper
- 1/2 pound sugar snap peas, strings removed
- 1/2 teaspoon dried rosemary, crushed

Put potatoes in a large pan, cover with water, and place over high heat. Boil potatoes about 15 minutes, or until tender when pierced with a fork. During the last 10 minutes that the potatoes are cooking, melt margarine in a large skillet. Add salt, pepper, and peas to margarine. Cook peas over high heat for 4 minutes, tossing frequently. Peas should be crisp-tender. Add cooked potatoes and rosemary to peas, then toss to coat.

Makes 7 (1/7 of recipe) servings
Preparation time: 15 minutes
Cooking time: 19 minutes

Nutrient Information (per serving):

Servings per recipe 7
Serving size 1/7 of recipe
Carbohydrate choices 1 1/2
Calories 131
Carbohydrate 22 grams
Protein 4 grams
Fat 3 grams
Saturated Fat 1 gram

Cholesterol 0
Sodium 383 milligrams
Dietary Fiber 3 grams
% calories from:
  Protein 12%
  Carbohydrate 67%
  Fat 21%

Food Exchanges: 1 1/2 starch

Greek Broiled Potatoes

"What I say is, if a man really likes potatoes, he must be a pretty decent sort of fellow."—A.A. Milne

S

6 medium baking potatoes

16-ounce can fat-free, reduced-sodium chicken broth

1 teaspoon salt

1/2 teaspoon coarse ground black pepper

1/2 teaspoon garlic powder

1/2 teaspoon onion powder

1/4 teaspoon paprika

3 tablespoons reduced-calorie margarine, melted

Preheat oven to 350°. Peel potatoes and cut in half lengthwise. Place flat side down in baking dish. Pour broth over potatoes. Sprinkle potatoes with salt, pepper, garlic powder, onion powder, and paprika. Bake for 1 hour, or until potatoes are tender when pierced with a fork. Brush with melted margarine and place 4 inches under broiler for 4 minutes or until crispy on top. Leave oven door cracked during broiling.

Makes 6 (1 potato) servings
Preparation time: 15 minutes
Cooking time: 1 hour and 4 minutes

Nutrient Information (per serving):

Servings per recipe 6

Serving size 1 potato

Carbohydrate choices 3

Calories 194

Carbohydrate 39 grams

Protein 5 grams

Fat 2 grams

Saturated Fat <1 gram

Cholesterol 0

Sodium 441 milligrams

Dietary Fiber 4 grams

% calories from:

Protein 10%

Carbohydrate 80%

Fat 9%

Food Exchanges: 2 starch, 1 vegetable

Crispy Oven "Fries"

Fries without the grease? It is possible—coating the potato wedges with cooking spray allows the seasonings to stick and the "fries" to turn crispy when baked.

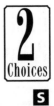

2 Choices

S

4 baking potatoes (about 2 pounds)
Cooking spray
1/2 cup grated Parmesan cheese
1/8 teaspoon cayenne pepper
1 1/2 teaspoons garlic salt

Preheat oven to 375°. Slice each potato lengthwise into 10 wedges, leaving skin on. Coat wedges with cooking spray. In a zip-top plastic bag, combine cheese, pepper, and garlic salt. Add half of potato wedges, seal bag, and shake to coat. Arrange potato wedges in a single layer on a baking sheet coated with cooking spray. Repeat procedure with remaining wedges. Bake for 15 minutes. Turn wedges over and continue baking for an additional 15 minutes, or until outside of potatoes are crispy and inside is tender when pierced with a fork.

Makes 8 (5 wedges) servings
Preparation time: 10 minutes
Baking time: 30 minutes

Nutrient Information (per serving):

Servings per recipe 8	Cholesterol 5 milligrams
Serving size 5 potato wedges	Sodium 510 milligrams
Carbohydrate choices 2	Dietary Fiber 3 grams
Calories 154	% calories from:
Carbohydrate 29 grams	Protein 13%
Protein 5 grams	Carbohydrate 75%
Fat 2 grams	Fat 12%
Saturated Fat 1 gram	

Food Exchanges: 2 starch

Garlic and Chive Mashed Potatoes

In years past, potatoes were thought to be poisonous and to cause a multitude of health problems. It wasn't until the mid-1800s that potatoes gained in popularity. Mashed potatoes are now an adored American side dish. Savor the mild onion-like flavor of chives mingled with the distinct flavor of garlic in this favorite.

4 potatoes, peeled and thinly sliced
4 cloves garlic, peeled
3 tablespoons reduced-calorie margarine
1/4 cup skim milk
1 1/2 tablespoons chopped fresh chives
1/2 teaspoon salt
1/8 teaspoon black pepper

Place potatoes and garlic in large pan, just cover with water, and bring to a boil over high heat. Reduce heat and boil gently for 15 minutes, or until potato slices break apart when pierced with a fork. Remove from heat and drain well, reserving garlic cloves along with potatoes. Beat potatoes and garlic with electric mixer until smooth. Add margarine and beat again. Add milk and whip until fluffy. Mix in chives, salt, and pepper and serve hot.

Makes 6 (1/2 cup) servings
Preparation time: 15 minutes
Cooking time: 15 minutes

Nutrient Information (per serving):

Servings per recipe 6

Serving size 1/2 cup

Carbohydrate choices 2 1/2

Calories 183

Carbohydrate 35 grams

Protein 4 grams

Fat 3 grams

Saturated Fat <1 gram

Cholesterol <1 milligram

Sodium 278 milligrams

Dietary Fiber 3 grams

% calories from:

Protein 9%

Carbohydrate 77%

Fat 15%

Food Exchanges: 2 starch, 1 vegetable

Sensational Stuffed Sweet Potatoes

More than just a sweet potato, this is a blending of harvest treasures—cranberries, apples, and walnuts enhanced by just a touch of brown sugar and cinnamon.

6 medium sweet potatoes

1/4 cup fresh cranberries

5 tablespoons reduced-calorie margarine

1 tablespoon brown sugar

1 teaspoon cinnamon

1/4 cup orange juice

1/2 apple, peeled, cored, and finely chopped

1/4 cup walnuts, finely chopped

Preheat oven to 400°. Place the sweet potatoes in a baking dish and bake for 20 minutes. Pierce potatoes with fork and continue baking 25 minutes, or until tender. Remove from oven and let cool slightly. Meanwhile, place the cranberries in a saucepan with enough water to cover berries. Bring to a boil and cook until the berries pop open, about 5 minutes; set aside. When potatoes are cool enough to touch, cut in half lengthwise, scoop out pulp, and set aside. Reserve the shells.

Reduce oven temperature to 325°. In a large bowl, mash the sweet potato pulp with a fork or potato masher (it does not need to be whipped). Mix in the margarine, brown sugar, and cinnamon. Stir in cranberries, orange juice, and apple. Place the mixture in the reserved shells, sprinkle with walnuts, and return to the oven. Bake until heated through, about 15 minutes.

Makes 6 (1 potato) servings
Preparation time: 15 minutes
Baking time: 60 minutes

Nutrient Information (per serving):

Servings per recipe 6	Cholesterol 0
Serving size 1 potato	Sodium 152 milligrams
Carbohydrate choices 3	Dietary Fiber 1 gram
Calories 252	% calories from:
Carbohydrate 41 grams	Protein 6%
Protein 4 grams	Carbohydrate 65%
Fat 8 grams	Fat 29%
Saturated Fat 1 gram	

Food Exchanges: 1 starch, 2 fruit, 1 fat

Green Bean Sauté

The delicate taste of thyme complements the tomatoes and onions in these green beans. If you prefer to use dried thyme, try 1/2 teaspoon instead of 1 teaspoon.

1 1/2 pounds fresh green beans, strings removed

3 tablespoons + 1 teaspoon reduced-calorie margarine

1 medium onion, coarsely chopped

1 teaspoon crushed garlic

1 teaspoon chopped fresh thyme

4 Roma tomatoes, peeled, seeded, and coarsely chopped

1/2 teaspoon salt

1/4 teaspoon black pepper

In a stockpot half filled with boiling water, blanch the beans for 8 minutes. Drain beans in colander and rinse with cold running water to stop the cooking process. Set beans aside.

Melt margarine in large skillet. Add onion and cook over medium heat until translucent. Stir in garlic, thyme, tomatoes, salt, and pepper. Cook for 1 minute. Add green beans and toss to coat. Heat thoroughly.

Makes 12 (1/2 cup) servings
Preparation time: 25 minutes

Nutrient Information (per serving):

Servings per recipe 12	Cholesterol 0
Serving size 1/2 cup	Sodium 128 milligrams
Carbohydrate choices 1/2	Dietary Fiber 1 gram
Calories 42	% calories from:
Carbohydrate 5 grams	Protein 10%
Protein 1 gram	Carbohydrate 48%
Fat 2 grams	Fat 43%
Saturated Fat <1 gram	

Food Exchanges: 1 vegetable, 1/2 fat

Spicy Three-Bean Combo

This is even more flavorful the next day, and it's quite versatile, too! In addition to a side dish, try this as a salad or a dip with tortilla chips.

15 1/2-ounce can red beans, rinsed and drained
15-ounce can Great Northern beans, rinsed and drained
15 1/2-ounce can black beans, rinsed and drained
4 Roma tomatoes, seeded and chopped
1 medium green pepper, seeded and chopped
1/2 cup chopped green onions (about 3 onions)
3/4 cup medium salsa
1/4 cup red-wine vinegar
2 tablespoons chopped fresh parsley
1/4 teaspoon salt
1/4 teaspoon black pepper

Place all ingredients in a large serving bowl and toss well. Cover and refrigerate at least 1 hour to allow flavors to blend.

Makes 15 (1/2 cup) servings
Preparation time: 15 minutes
Chilling time: 1 hour

Nutrient Information (per serving):

Servings per recipe 15	Cholesterol 0
Serving size 1/2 cup	Sodium 183 milligrams
Carbohydrate choices 1 1/2	Dietary Fiber 3 grams
Calories 117	% calories from:
Carbohydrate 20 grams	Protein 24%
Protein 7 grams	Carbohydrate 68%
Fat 1 gram	Fat 9%
Saturated Fat <1 gram	

Food Exchanges: 1 starch, 1 vegetable

Mom's Old-Fashioned Baked Beans

This recipe, passed down to Tami by her mother, is a family favorite at summer cookouts. It is also a nice accompaniment to the Gourmet Peppered-Turkey Bagel Sandwich (page 98).

2 1 pound 13-ounce cans pinto beans
1 teaspoon salt
1/2 teaspoon black pepper
1 tablespoon instant chopped onion
1 1/2 cups ketchup
1/2 tablespoon brown mustard
1 tablespoon Worcestershire sauce
1/2 tablespoon Red Hot sauce
2 tablespoons molasses
Cooking spray
4 strips bacon, cooked, drained, and crumbled

Preheat oven to 375°. In a large bowl, stir together first 9 ingredients. Place in large casserole dish coated with cooking spray. Sprinkle with bacon. Cover and bake for one hour.

Makes 16 (1/2 cup) servings
Preparation time: 10 minutes
Baking time: 1 hour

Nutrient Information (per serving):

Servings per recipe 16	Cholesterol 1 milligram
Serving size 1/2 cup	Sodium 820 milligrams
Carbohydrate choices 1 1/2	Dietary Fiber 4 grams
Calories 125	% calories from:
Carbohydrate 23 grams	Protein 19%
Protein 6 grams	Carbohydrate 74%
Fat 1 gram	Fat 7%
Saturated Fat <1 gram	

Food Exchanges: 1 starch, 1 vegetable

Great Northern Beans with Garlic and Rosemary

A pungent accompaniment filled with fiber. Try serving alongside a grilled chicken breast or pork chop.

F

2 15-ounce cans Great Northern beans, rinsed and drained
1/3 cup reduced-sodium, fat-free chicken bouillon
1 teaspoon crushed garlic
1/2 teaspoon crushed dried rosemary
2 dashes cayenne pepper

Place all ingredients in a medium pan and cook over low-medium heat for 20 minutes; stir periodically.

Makes 8 (1/2) cup servings
Preparation time: 5 minutes
Cooking time: 20 minutes

Nutrient Information (per serving):

Servings per recipe 8	Cholesterol <1 milligram
Serving size 1/2 cup	Sodium 165 milligrams
Carbohydrate choices 1 1/2	Dietary Fiber 5 grams
Calories 133	% calories from:
Carbohydrate 23 grams	Protein 25%
Protein 8 grams	Carbohydrate 72%
Fat <1 gram	Fat 3%
Saturated Fat <1 gram	

Food Exchanges: 1 starch, 1 vegetable, 1 very lean meat

Savory Black Bean and Shoepeg Corn Salsa

Use as spicy side dish to accompany grilled or baked fish.

2 jalapeno peppers, seeded and diced
1 red bell pepper, seeded and diced
15-ounce can black beans, rinsed and drained
11-ounce can shoepeg corn, rinsed and drained
1/3 cup chopped fresh parsley
1/4 cup diced purple onion
1/4 cup chopped green onions
1/3 cup fresh-squeezed lime juice
2 tablespoons corn oil
1 tablespoon ground cumin
1/4 teaspoon salt
1/2 teaspoon coarse ground black pepper
1 cup seeded, chopped Roma tomatoes

In a large bowl, combine jalapeno pepper, red pepper, beans, corn, parsley, purple onion, and green onions. In a small bowl mix together lime juice, oil, cumin, salt, and black pepper. Pour over bean mixture and toss well. Cover and refrigerate at least 3 hours to allow flavors to blend. Just before serving, toss in tomatoes.

Makes 14 (1/2 cup) servings
Preparation time: 15 minutes
Chilling time: 3 hours

Nutrient Information (per serving):

Servings per recipe 14

Serving size 1/2 cup

Carbohydrate choices 1

Calories 61

Carbohydrate 11 grams

Protein 2 grams

Fat <1 gram

Saturated Fat <1 gram

Cholesterol 0

Sodium 283 milligrams

Dietary Fiber 3 grams

% calories from:

  Protein 13%

  Carbohydrate 72%

  Fat 15%

Food Exchanges: 2 vegetable

Cherry Walnut Brown Rice

A variety of dried fruits are growing in popularity. Look for dried cherries in the produce section or where dried fruits are located in your supermarket.

3 tablespoons reduced-calorie margarine

1 medium onion, finely chopped

1 cup finely chopped celery

4 cups hot, cooked brown rice

3/4 cup dried bing cherries

1/4 cup toasted, chopped walnuts

3 green onions, diced

1/4 teaspoon salt

1/8 teaspoon black pepper

Melt margarine in a large nonstick skillet over medium heat. Add onion and celery and cook until onion is translucent. Stir in brown rice, cherries, walnuts, onions, salt, and pepper. Combine well; heat through.

Makes 10 (1/2 cup) servings
Preparation time: 10 minutes

Nutrient Information (per serving):

Servings per recipe 10

Serving size 1/2 cup

Carbohydrate choices 2

Calories 164

Carbohydrate 29 grams

Protein 3 grams

Fat 4 grams

Saturated Fat <1 gram

Cholesterol 0

Sodium 112 milligrams

Dietary Fiber 1 gram

% calories from:

Protein 7%

Carbohydrate 71%

Fat 22%

Food Exchanges: 1 starch, 1 fruit, 1 fat

Seasoned Wild Rice with Mushrooms

Wild rice is actually the seed from a wild grass that grows in the northern United States. Its nutritional composition is closer to wheat than to rice.

4 cups water

1 teaspoon salt

3 1/2 cups instant long grain and wild rice

2 tablespoons reduced-calorie margarine

8-ounce package fresh mushrooms, thinly sliced

1/4 cup diced green onion

1/4 cup white cooking wine

3/4 cup reduced-sodium, fat-free beef bouillon

2 tablespoons reduced-calorie margarine

Place water and salt in a large pan, stir in rice, and bring to a boil. Cover and reduce heat to a low-medium. Cook rice for 5 minutes, or until the water is absorbed and the rice is fluffy.

Meanwhile, in a small skillet, melt 2 tablespoons margarine over medium heat. Add mushrooms and onions and cook for 5 minutes. Stir in wine and bouillon. Add remaining margarine and sautéed vegetables with liquid to the cooked rice and toss well.

Makes 7 (1 cup) servings
Preparation time: 5 minutes
Cooking time: 20 minutes

Nutrient Information (per serving):

Servings per recipe 7
Serving size 1 cup
Carbohydrate choices 3
Calories 236
Carbohydrate 44 grams
Protein 6 grams
Fat 4 grams
Saturated Fat 1 gram

Cholesterol 0
Sodium 385 milligrams
Dietary Fiber 1 gram
% calories from:
  Protein 10%
  Carbohydrate 75%
  Fat 15%

Food Exchanges: 3 starch

Angel Hair Pasta, Mediterranean-Style

2 Choices

This colorful side dish can double as a refreshing entrée or luncheon.

4 cups seeded and chopped Roma tomatoes
1 tablespoon olive oil
1 tablespoon red wine vinegar
2 tablespoons chopped fresh basil
1/4 teaspoon salt
1/8 teaspoon crushed red pepper flakes
1 teaspoon crushed garlic
2 tablespoons capers
4 cups cooked angel hair pasta, cooled
1/4 cup (1 ounce) crumbled feta cheese
1 tablespoon finely chopped black olives

In a large bowl, stir together tomatoes, olive oil, vinegar, basil, salt, red pepper, garlic, and capers. Refrigerate for 15 minutes to allow flavors to blend. Place pasta in serving dish and spoon tomato mixture over it. Sprinkle with feta cheese and chopped black olives.

Makes 7 (I cup) servings
Preparation time: 15 minutes
Chilling time: 15 minutes

Nutrient Information (per serving):

Servings per recipe 7
Serving size I cup
Carbohydrate choices 2
Calories 164
Carbohydrate 27 grams
Protein 5 grams
Fat 4 grams
Saturated Fat I gram

Cholesterol 4 milligrams
Sodium 221 milligrams
Dietary Fiber I gram
% calories from:
    Protein 12%
    Carbohydrate 66%
    Fat 22%

Food Exchanges: 2 starch

Summer Squash Sauté

The yellow squash is one of several types of "summer" squash. To maintain the crisp-tenderness of the squash, serve immediately.

5 teaspoons reduced-calorie margarine
Cooking spray
4 small yellow summer squash, sliced in 1/2-inch slices
I small onion, sliced and separated into rings
4 1/2-ounce can chopped green chilies, drained
1/4 teaspoon garlic salt

Melt margarine over medium heat in a large nonstick skillet coated with cooking spray. Add squash and onions. Cook, stirring periodically, for 10 minutes. Add green chilies and garlic salt. Cook for an additional 5 minutes, or until squash is tender when pierced with a fork.

Makes 5 (1 cup) servings
Preparation time: 5 minutes
Cooking time: 15 minutes

Nutrient Information (per serving):

Servings per recipe 5	Cholesterol 0
Serving size 1 cup	Sodium 242 milligrams
Carbohydrate choices 1	Dietary Fiber 3 grams
Calories 62	% calories from:
Carbohydrate 9 grams	Protein 13%
Protein 2 grams	Carbohydrate 58%
Fat 2 grams	Fat 29%
Saturated Fat <1 gram	

Food Exchanges: 2 vegetable

Brown-Sugar Butternut Squash

$1\frac{1}{2}$ Choices

The butternut squash may also be referred to as a "winter squash." If you want to prepare this a bit ahead of serving time, leave off the walnuts and brown sugar and hold squash mixture in a warm oven. Just before delivering to the table, add walnuts and brown sugar and place under broiler as directed.

1 butternut squash

3 tablespoons reduced-calorie margarine

1/4 teaspoon salt

Cooking spray

2 tablespoons finely chopped walnuts

2 tablespoons brown sugar

Peel squash, cut in half, and remove seeds. Chop into 1-inch cubes and place in pan. Add water to pan to just cover squash. Place lid on pan and cook over medium heat until squash is tender, about 25 minutes. Drain water. Using an electric mixer, whip squash until smooth. Add margarine and salt and whip again. Spoon into baking dish coated with cooking spray, then sprinkle with walnuts and brown sugar. Place under broiler for 3 minutes, or until brown sugar is bubbly. Take care not to burn walnuts.

Makes 4 (1/2 cup) servings
Preparation time: 15 minutes
Cooking time: 30 minutes

Nutrient Information (per serving):

Servings per recipe 4	Cholesterol 0
Serving size 1/2 cup	Sodium 235 milligrams
Carbohydrate choices 1 1/2	Dietary Fiber 3 grams
Calories 135	% calories from:
Carbohydrate 16 grams	Protein 6%
Protein 2 grams	Carbohydrate 47%
Fat 7 grams	Fat 47%
Saturated Fat 1 gram	

Food Exchanges: 1 starch, 1 fat

Country Corn Pudding

Use fresh corn in this side dish for the finest flavor. If a deep baking dish is used, increase the cooking time as needed.

3/4 cup liquid egg substitute

2 cups skim milk

4 tablespoons all-purpose flour

2 tablespoons sugar

1 teaspoon salt

2 cups corn

Cooking spray

3 tablespoons reduced-calorie stick margarine

Preheat oven to 350°. Place egg substitute, milk, flour, sugar, and salt in a mixing bowl and combine using a whisk. Stir in corn. Pour in a shallow casserole dish coated with cooking spray. Dot top with margarine. Bake for 15 minutes. Stir, then return to oven and bake an additional 20 minutes, or until a knife inserted into the center of pudding comes out clean.

Makes 6 (1/2 cup) servings
Preparation time: 5 minutes
Baking time: 35 minutes

Nutrient Information (per serving):

Servings per recipe 6	Cholesterol 2 milligrams
Serving size 1/2 cup	Sodium 555 milligrams
Carbohydrate choices 2	Dietary Fiber 1 gram
Calories 168	% calories from:
Carbohydrate 24 grams	Protein 21%
Protein 9 grams	Carbohydrate 57%
Fat 4 grams	Fat 21%
Saturated Fat <1 gram	

Food Exchanges: 1 starch, 2 vegetable, 1/2 lean meat

Quick Broccoli Parmesano

A new rendition of broccoli with cheese!

3 tablespoons reduced-calorie margarine
1 onion, finely chopped
2 pounds broccoli florets
2 cups sliced fresh mushrooms
2 teaspoons lemon juice
1/2 teaspoon salt
1/4 teaspoon black pepper
1/8 teaspoon garlic powder
1/4 cup fresh grated Parmesan cheese

Melt margarine in a large nonstick skillet over medium-high heat. Add onion and cook, stirring frequently, until onion is translucent. Add broccoli and cook until broccoli is crisp-tender, about 7 minutes. Add mushrooms and cook 3 more minutes. Sprinkle vegetables with lemon juice, salt, pepper, and garlic powder. Toss to coat. Place in serving dish and top with Parmesan cheese.

Makes 8 (1 cup) servings
Preparation time: 20 minutes

Nutrient Information (per serving):

Servings per recipe 8

Serving size 1 cup

Carbohydrate choices 1

Calories 83

Carbohydrate 9 grams

Protein 5 grams

Fat 3 grams

Saturated Fat <1 gram

Cholesterol 2 milligrams

Sodium 275 milligrams

Dietary Fiber 4 grams

% calories from:

    Protein 24%

    Carbohydrate 43%

    Fat 33%

Food Exchanges: 2 vegetable, 1 fat

Dilly-Lemon Glazed Baby Carrots

$\frac{1}{2}$ Choice

The delicate taste of dill intermingled with a lemony tartness provides a simple, yet splendid complement to the sweet flavor of carrots.

16-ounce bag baby carrots

2 tablespoons fresh-squeezed lemon juice

2/3 cup water

2 teaspoons cornstarch

2 teaspoons reduced-calorie margarine

1/2 teaspoon dried dillweed

1/4 teaspoon lemon pepper

1/4 teaspoon salt

Place carrots in a steamer pan over 2 inches boiling water. Cover and steam 10 minutes, or until carrots are crisp-tender when pierced with a fork. Transfer carrots to a serving dish, cover, and keep warm.

In a small saucepan combine lemon juice, water, and cornstarch. Whisk until cornstarch is dissolved. Place pan over medium heat and cook until thickened, whisking constantly. Add margarine, dillweed, lemon pepper, and salt. Cook another 3 minutes, stirring constantly. Pour glaze over carrots and toss to coat.

Makes 8 (1/2 cup) servings
Preparation time: 15 minutes

Nutrient Information (per serving):

Servings per recipe 8	Cholesterol 0
Serving size 1/2 cup	Sodium 115 milligrams
Carbohydrate choices 1/2	Dietary Fiber <1 gram
Calories 37	% calories from:
Carbohydrate 6 grams	Protein 11%
Protein <1 gram	Carbohydrate 65%
Fat 1 gram	Fat 24%
Saturated Fat <1 gram	

Food Exchanges: 1 vegetable

Tangy Marinated Carrot Coins

A colorful sweet 'n sour side dish that uniquely incorporates canned tomato soup as the marinade's base!

1½ Choices

F

- 6 cups sliced carrot coins, cooked until just tender
- 1 large onion, sliced into rings and separated
- 1/2 yellow pepper, diced
- 1/2 green pepper, diced

Marinade:
- 10 3/4-ounce can reduced-sodium, reduced-fat tomato soup
- 1 cup white vinegar
- 1 teaspoon Worcestershire sauce
- 1/4 cup canola oil
- 10 packets aspartame sweetener
- 1 teaspoon ground mustard
- 1 teaspoon black pepper
- 1/2 teaspoon salt

Combine carrot coins, onion rings, and diced peppers in a serving dish and set aside. Combine all marinade ingredients in a large jar and screw lid on tightly. Shake until well mixed. Pour over vegetables, cover, and marinate 8 hours, or overnight, in refrigerator.

Makes 8 (1 cup) servings
Preparation time: 20 minutes
Chilling time: 8 hours

Nutrient Information (per serving):

Servings per recipe 8

Serving size 1 cup

Carbohydrate choices 1 1/2

Calories 137

Carbohydrate 20 grams

Protein 3 grams

Fat 5 grams

Saturated Fat <1 gram

Cholesterol 0

Sodium 246 milligrams

Dietary Fiber 5 grams

% calories from:

   Protein 9%

   Carbohydrate 58%

   Fat 33%

Food Exchanges: 1 starch, 1 vegetable, 1 fat

Dilled Peas, Carrots, and Pearl Onions

$\frac{1}{2}$ Choice

A showy side dish! Dill complements each vegetable's flavor while walnuts add crunch.

   15-ounce can small very young peas, rinsed and drained

   15-ounce can baby carrots, rinsed and drained

   15-ounce jar pearl onions, drained

   3 tablespoons reduced-calorie margarine

   1 teaspoon dried dillweed

   1/4 cup walnut pieces

Put peas, carrots, and onions each in 3 separate pans and warm over low-medium heat. May add a small amount of water to each pan to prevent sticking. Meanwhile, melt margarine in a small saucepan. Add dillweed and walnut pieces. Cook over medium heat for 3 minutes, stirring frequently. Drain vegetables and place in mounds, by vegetable, on a serving platter. Drizzle with the walnut/margarine mixture and serve.

Makes 11 (1/2 cup) servings

Preparation time: 10 minutes

Nutrient Information (per serving):

Servings per recipe 11
Serving size 1/2 cup
Carbohydrate choices 1/2
Calories 71
Carbohydrate 8 grams
Protein 3 grams
Fat 3 grams
Saturated Fat <1 gram

Cholesterol 0
Sodium 304 milligrams
Dietary Fiber 3 grams
% calories from:
   Protein 17%
   Carbohydrate 45%
   Fat 38%

Food Exchanges: 2 vegetable, 1/2 fat

Basil and Chive Tomato Bake

As Alice Walters so wisely stated, "Once you taste a tomato in
the summer, you won't eat a tomato in the winter." Juicy tomatoes fresh from the garden certainly lend the best flavor to this
delightful side dish.

Cooking spray

3 cups garlic croutons

6 large ripe tomatoes, sliced 1/2-inch thick

1/2 teaspoon coarse ground black pepper

2 cups shredded, reduced-fat mozzarella cheese

2 tablespoons dried basil

1 tablespoon dried chives

3 tablespoons canola oil

1/4 cup red wine vinegar

Preheat oven to 350°. Coat a 9"x 13" baking dish with cooking
spray and cover bottom of dish with croutons. Overlap tomatoes
on top of croutons. Sprinkle tomatoes with pepper, then cheese,
basil, and chives. Bake uncovered for 10 minutes. Remove from
oven and drizzle with oil, then vinegar. Return to oven and cook
uncovered an additional 10 minutes.

Makes 8 (1/8 of casserole) servings
Preparation time: 10 minutes
Baking time: 20 minutes

Nutrient Information (per serving):

Servings per recipe 8

Serving size 1/8 of casserole

Carbohydrate choices 1

Calories 191

Carbohydrate 14 grams

Protein 9 grams

Fat 11 grams

Saturated Fat 3 grams

Cholesterol 16 milligrams

Sodium 219 milligrams

Dietary Fiber 2 grams

% calories from:

  Protein 19%

  Carbohydrate 29%

Fat 52%

Food Exchanges: 2 vegetables, 1 medium-fat meat, 1 fat

Corny Tomato Boats

*Roma tomatoes make a creative serving dish for this
colorful combination!*

1½
Choices

10 large Roma tomatoes

15 1/4-ounce can corn, rinsed and drained

15 1/2-ounce can black beans, rinsed and drained

4 1/2-ounce can chopped green chilies

1 tablespoon corn oil

3 tablespoons red wine vinegar

1 teaspoon dried chopped parsley

1/2 teaspoon dried oregano

1/4 teaspoon salt

1/8 teaspoon black pepper

Cut tomatoes in half lengthwise, scoop out seeds and pulp, place
cut-side down on paper towels to drain for 15 minutes, then
refrigerate until ready to fill. Meanwhile, combine corn, beans,
and chilies in a large bowl and set aside. Place oil, vinegar, parsley, oregano, salt, and pepper in a jar and cover tightly with lid.

Shake to combine. Pour over corn mixture and stir to coat. Refrigerate for at least 1 hour to allow flavors to blend.

Spoon 1/8 cup corn mixture into each tomato boat and refrigerate until serving time.

Makes 10 (2 boat) servings
Preparation time: 20 minutes
Chilling time: 1 hour

Nutrient Information (per serving):

Servings per recipe 10
Serving size 2 boats
Carbohydrate choices 1 1/2
Calories 130
Carbohydrate 22 grams
Protein 6 grams
Fat 2 grams
Saturated Fat <1 gram

Cholesterol 0
Sodium 106 milligrams
Dietary Fiber 3 grams
% calories from:
  Protein 18%
  Carbohydrate 68%
  Fat 14%

Food Exchanges: 1 starch, 1 vegetable

Tangy Cauliflower Toss

Red wine vinegar and lemon pepper add tang to this simple vegetable side dish.

1 Choice

1 medium head cauliflower, broken into florets
2 tablespoons canola oil
2 tablespoons red wine vinegar
1/2 teaspoon crushed garlic
1/4 teaspoon salt
1/4 teaspoon lemon pepper

Put cauliflower florets in a steamer pan over 2 inches boiling water. Cover and steam 7 minutes, or until tender when pierced with a fork. Meanwhile, combine oil, vinegar, garlic, salt, and lemon pepper in a saucepan and warm over medium heat. Place cauliflower in serving dish, drizzle with oil mixture, and toss gently to coat.

Makes 4 (1 cup) servings
Preparation time: 12 minutes

Nutrient Information (per serving):

Servings per recipe 4
Serving size 1 cup
Carbohydrate choices 1
Calories 111
Carbohydrate 9 grams
Protein 3 grams
Fat 7 grams
Saturated Fat <1 gram

Cholesterol 0
Sodium 191 milligrams
Dietary Fiber 4 grams
% calories from:
  Protein 11%
  Carbohydrate 32%
  Fat 57%

Food Exchanges: 2 vegetable, 1 fat

Grilled Eggplant Oregano

$\frac{1}{2}$ Choice

As Julia Child notes, "Eggplant is a handsome vegetable indeed, with its green cap and purple skin." Choose an eggplant that is firm, unblemished, and heavy for its size. Store in a plastic bag in the refrigerator for up to five days.

> 1 large eggplant
> 3 tablespoons olive oil
> 1/2 teaspoon crushed dried oregano
> 1/2 teaspoon salt

Slice eggplant into 1/2-inch-thick rings. Brush both sides of each ring with olive oil, then sprinkle lightly with oregano and salt. Place eggplant on grill over hot coals and cook until tender, but not mushy, about 3 minutes per side. Turn once during cooking.

Makes 5 (2 slice) servings
Preparation time: 10 minutes
Cooking time: 6 minutes

Nutrient Information (per serving):

Servings per recipe 5

Serving size 2 slices

Carbohydrate choices 1/2

Calories 100

Carbohydrate 6 grams

Protein 1 gram

Fat 8 grams

Saturated Fat 1 gram

Cholesterol 0

Sodium 235 milligrams

Dietary Fiber 2 grams

% calories from:

Protein 4%

Carbohydrate 24%

Fat 72%

Food Exchanges: 2 vegetable, 1 fat

Pineapple Glazed Beets

"The discovery of a new dish does more for the happiness of mankind than the discovery of a star."—Brillat-Savarin
You will be happy that you discovered this unique fruit and vegetable combination!

> 20-ounce can crushed pineapple, packed in juice
>
> 1/2 teaspoon brown sugar substitute
>
> 1/2 teaspoon allspice
>
> 2 tablespoons reduced-calorie margarine
>
> 2 tablespoons lemon juice
>
> 2 15 1/4-ounce cans sliced beets, drained

Drain pineapple, reserving juice. In a large saucepan, whisk together brown sugar substitute, allspice, and reserved pineapple juice. Cook over medium heat until mixture is warm. Stir in margarine and lemon juice. Add beets and pineapple to glaze. Cook over medium heat for 5 minutes, or until beets are warm.

Makes 8 (1/2 cup) servings
Preparation time: 15 minutes

Nutrient Information (per serving):

Servings per recipe 8

Serving size 1/2 cup

Carbohydrate choices 1

Calories 78

Carbohydrate 14 grams

Protein 1 gram

Fat 2 grams

Saturated Fat <1 gram

Cholesterol 0

Sodium 332 milligrams

Dietary Fiber 2 grams

% calories from:

Protein 5%

Carbohydrate 72%

Fat 18%

Food Exchanges: 1 starch

Creole Cabbage

Best if served immediately after cooking to maintain the crisp cabbage texture.

$\frac{1}{2}$ Choice

1 tablespoon reduced-calorie margarine

4 cups shredded cabbage

1/4 cup chopped onion

1/4 cup finely diced celery

1/4 cup chopped green pepper

1 cup canned diced tomatoes, drained

3/4 teaspoon salt

1/8 teaspoon black pepper

1/4 teaspoon garlic powder

4 dashes cayenne pepper

Melt margarine in a large nonstick skillet over medium heat. Add remaining ingredients and cook 15 minutes, or until cabbage is crisp-tender.

Makes 5 (1/2 cup) servings
Preparation time: 10 minutes
Cooking time: 15 minutes

Nutrient Information (per serving):

Servings per recipe 5

Serving size 1/2 cup

Carbohydrate choices 1/2

Calories 41

Carbohydrate 7 grams

Protein 1 gram

Fat 1 gram

Saturated Fat <1 gram

Cholesterol 0

Sodium 395 milligrams

Dietary Fiber 2 grams

% calories from:

Protein 10%

Carbohydrate 68%

Fat 22%

Food Exchanges: 2 vegetable

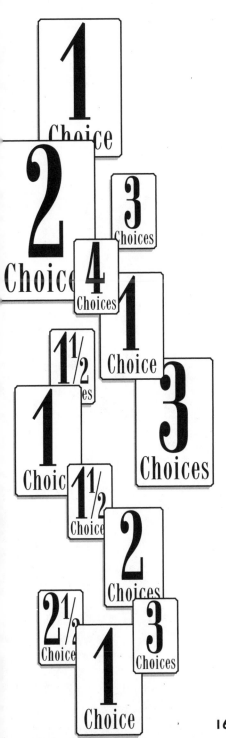

Desserts

Kahlua Ice Cream Dessert

The ice cream for this recipe can be quickly softened by thawing in the microwave on low.

2 cups reduced-fat chocolate-flavored vanilla wafer crumbs
3 tablespoons reduced-calorie stick margarine, melted
Cooking spray
12 1/4-ounce jar fat-free caramel ice cream topping
1/4 cup Kahlua
1/2 gallon reduced-fat, no-sugar-added vanilla ice cream, softened
1/4 cup reduced-fat chocolate-flavored vanilla wafer crumbs

In a mixing bowl, stir together 2 cups crumbs and margarine. Press crumb mixture into bottom of 9" x 13" pan coated with cooking spray. Drizzle caramel topping over crust. Freeze for 1/2 hour, or until crust hardens.

In a large bowl, mix Kahlua into softened ice cream. Spread over frozen crumb crust. Sprinkle with remaining 1/4 cup crumbs. Return to freezer for at least 2 hours to allow ice cream to harden.

Makes 15 (1 square) servings
Preparation time: 20 minutes
Freezing time: 2 1/2 hours

Nutrient Information (per serving):

Servings per recipe 15	Cholesterol 0
Serving size 1 square	Sodium 212 milligrams
Carbohydrate choices 2 1/2	Dietary Fiber 1 gram
Calories 204	% calories from:
Carbohydrate 35 grams	Protein 8%
Protein 4 grams	Carbohydrate 69%
Fat 3 grams	Fat 13%
Saturated Fat <1 gram	Alcohol: 10%

Food Exchanges: 2 starch, 1/2 other carbohydrates

Triple Chocolate Parfait

Chocolate-flavored vanilla wafers, vanilla fudge swirl ice cream, and chocolate liqueur are the three chocolates in these pretty parfaits.

$2\frac{1}{2}$ Choices

48 reduced-fat chocolate-flavored vanilla wafer cookies

4 cups no-sugar-added vanilla fudge swirl ice cream (or chocolate ice cream)

1/2 cup chocolate liqueur

1/2 cup light whipped topping

In each of 8 parfait glasses layer 3 vanilla wafers, 1/4 cup ice cream, then 1 1/2 teaspoons liqueur. Repeat layers. Top each parfait with 1 tablespoon whipped topping. Freeze until serving time.

Makes 8 servings
Preparation time: 15 minutes

Nutrient Information (per serving):

Servings per recipe 8
Serving size 1 parfait
Carbohydrate choices 2 1/2
Calories 235
Carbohydrate 38 grams
Protein 5 grams
Fat 7 grams
Saturated Fat 3 grams

Cholesterol 15 milligrams
Sodium 156 milligrams
Dietary Fiber <1 gram
% calories from:
  Protein 8%
  Carbohydrate 64%
  Fat 26%
  Alcohol: 2%

Food Exchanges: 2 starch, 1 fat

Summer Strawberry Mousse

"Doubtless God could have made a better berry, but doubtless God never did."—William Butler

3 cups sliced frozen strawberries, no sugar added, thawed
4 teaspoons unflavored gelatin
1/4 cup warm water
1/2 cup powdered sugar
4 teaspoons lemon juice
12-ounce carton light whipped topping

Place strawberries in food processor or blender and process until smooth. Strain strawberry pulp through a sieve, pressing pulp with spoon. Set strained pulp aside and discard seeds remaining in sieve.

Combine gelatin and water in top of double boiler. Place over 2 inches boiling water and stir to dissolve gelatin. Remove from heat. To strawberry pulp, add dissolved gelatin, powdered sugar, and lemon juice; stir quickly to combine. With wire whisk, fold in whipped topping. Spoon into a 9" x 13" pan. Cover and freeze until consistency of frozen whipped topping, about 3 hours. Thaw slightly before serving and scoop into bowls with ice cream scoop.

Makes 10 (1/2 cup) servings
Preparation time: 15 minutes
Freezing time: 3 hours

Nutrient Information (per serving):

Servings per recipe 10

Serving size 1/2 cup

Carbohydrate choices 1 1/2

Calories 112

Carbohydrate 18 grams

Protein <1 gram

Fat 4 grams

Saturated Fat 4 grams

Cholesterol 0

Sodium 2 milligrams

Dietary Fiber 1 gram

% calories from:

  Protein 4%

  Carbohydrate 64%

  Fat 32%

Food Exchanges: 1 starch, 1 fat

Banana-Pineapple Confection

Almond extract complements the natural sweetness of the pineapple and banana in this thick and creamy confection. Serve in sherbet dishes and top with a maraschino cherry.

2 20-ounce cans crushed pineapple, packed in juice

4 peeled bananas

1 teaspoon almond extract

Pour pineapple and juice into shallow container. Put whole bananas on cookie sheet. Place pineapple and bananas in freezer and freeze for 3 hours, or until pineapple is just slightly slushy. Place frozen pineapple and bananas in blender along with almond extract; blend until thick and creamy (may have to blend in 2 batches if blender container is small). Serve immediately.

Makes 13 (1/2 cup) servings
Preparation time: 5 minutes
Freezing time: 3 hours

Nutrient Information (per serving):

Servings per recipe 13

Serving size 1/2 cup

Carbohydrate choices 1

Calories 69

Carbohydrate 15 grams

Protein 1 gram

Fat <1 gram

Saturated Fat <1 gram

Cholesterol 0

Sodium 1 milligram

Dietary Fiber 1 gram

% calories from:

Protein 6%

Carbohydrate 87%

Fat 7%

Food Exchanges: 1 fruit

Thumbprint Cookies

An inviting cookie with a hint of almond flavor. For a colorful tray of cookies, use a variety of fruit spreads to fill the thumbprints.

1 Choice

8-ounce package Sweet 'n Low low-fat white cake mix

3 tablespoons unsweetened orange juice

1/2 teaspoon almond extract

Cooking spray

5 teaspoons blueberry 100% fruit spread

Preheat oven to 350°. Place cake mix in a medium mixing bowl. Add orange juice and almond extract. Using an electric mixer, whip on low setting. As a dough begins to form, increase mixer to medium setting and beat for 2 minutes, or until a smooth dough is formed. Coat hands with cooking spray. Roll dough into 1-inch balls, and place on a baking sheet coated with cooking spray. Press center of each cookie with thumb. Fill thumbprint with 1/4 teaspoon blueberry spread. Bake for 10 minutes (cookies will turn light golden). Remove from baking sheet and cool on wire rack.

Makes 20 (1 cookie) servings
Preparation time: 10 minutes
Baking time: 10 minutes per pan

Nutrient Information (per serving):

Servings per recipe 20

Serving size 1 cookie

Carbohydrate choices 1

Calories 53

Carbohydrate 10 grams

Protein 1 gram

Fat 1 gram

Saturated Fat <1 gram

Cholesterol 0

Sodium 9 milligrams

Dietary Fiber <1 gram

% calories from:

Protein 8%

Carbohydrate 75%

Fat 17%

Food Exchanges: 1 fruit

Easy Refrigerator Bars

Orange juice and cinnamon add zip to these chewy bars.

1/2 cup reduced-fat chunky peanut butter

1/4 cup unsweetened orange juice

2 tablespoons honey

1/4 teaspoon ground cinnamon

3 cups crushed bran flake cereal

1/4 cup chopped raisins

1/4 cup chopped unsweetened dates

Cooking spray

In a large bowl, stir together peanut butter, orange juice, honey, and cinnamon. Mix in cereal, raisins, and dates. Press into an 8" x 8" pan coated with cooking spray and refrigerate for 2 hours.

Makes 16 (2 inch) bars
Preparation time: 10 minutes
Chilling time: 2 hours

Nutrient Information (per serving):

Servings per recipe 16
Serving size 1 (2 inch) bar
Carbohydrate choices 1 1/2
Calories 103
Carbohydrate 16 grams
Protein 3 grams
Fat 3 grams
Saturated Fat <1 gram

Cholesterol 0
Sodium 121 milligrams
Dietary Fiber 2 grams
% calories from:
　Protein 12%
　Carbohydrate 62%
　Fat 26%

Food Exchanges: 1 starch, 1/2 fruit

No-Bake Peanut Butter Cookies

No hassle and no baking required! Ready to eat
in just 15 minutes!

　1 cup powdered skim milk
　1 cup reduced-fat peanut butter
　2 tablespoons honey
　1/8 cup finely crushed chocolate graham crackers

In a large bowl, mix together powdered milk, peanut butter, and honey. Roll dough into 32 1-inch balls (dough will crumble easily). Put chocolate graham cracker crumbs in a shallow dish and roll each cookie ball in crumbs to lightly coat. Best if served same day.

Makes 32 (1-inch) cookies
Preparation time: 15 minutes

Servings per recipe 32

Serving size 1 cookie

Carbohydrate choices 1/2

Calories 67

Carbohydrate 7 grams

Protein 3 grams

Fat 3 grams

Saturated Fat <1 gram

Cholesterol <1 milligram

Sodium 80 milligrams

Dietary Fiber <1 gram

% calories from:

Protein 18%

Carbohydrate 42%

Fat 40%

Food Exchanges: 1/2 starch

Cream-Filled Chocolate Cupcakes

$1\frac{1}{2}$
Choices

Decadent chocolate cake with white chocolate cream cheese center.

8-ounce package Sweet 'n Low chocolate cake mix

2/3 cup water

Cooking spray

1/8 cup white chocolate chips

4 ounces reduced-fat cream cheese

1/8 cup sugar

1 teaspoon vanilla extract

1 teaspoon liquid egg substitute

Preheat oven to 375°. In a large mixing bowl, combine cake mix and half the water. Using an electric mixer, beat on medium for 3 minutes. Add remaining water and beat an additional 3 minutes. Spoon batter evenly into 12 muffin cups lined with paper baking cups and coated with cooking spray.

Melt white chocolate chips in double boiler pan over 2 inches boiling water. Meanwhile, in a medium mixing bowl, combine cream cheese and sugar. Beat with an electric mixer until fluffy. Mix in vanilla extract and egg substitute. Whip melted chocolate into cream cheese. Carefully spoon a dollop of cream cheese mixture into center of each cupcake. Bake for 20 minutes, or until centers of cupcakes are set. Cool 10 minutes in pans, then remove to wire racks to finish cooling. To preserve moistness, refrigerate if not served within 2 hours.

Makes 12 (1 cupcake) servings
Preparation time: 15 minutes
Baking time: 20 minutes

Nutrient Information (per serving):

Servings per recipe 12

Serving size 1 cupcake

Carbohydrate choices 1 1/2

Calories 120

Carbohydrate 19 grams

Protein 2 grams

Fat 4 grams

Saturated Fat 2 grams

Cholesterol 4 milligrams

Sodium 71 milligrams

Dietary Fiber 1 gram

% calories from:

Protein 7%

Carbohydrate 63%

Fat 30%

Food Exchanges: 1 starch, 1 fat

Orange Delight Dessert Loaf

A delightfully moist dessert loaf that boasts a mild orange flavor. Allow to cool completely for easier slicing. It's especially good drizzled with Raspberry-Orange Sauce (page 192). Or, try a dollop of light whipped topping with fresh blueberries or raspberries.

3/4 cup sugar

2 tablespoons reduced-calorie margarine

1 egg

3/4 cup skim milk

3/4 cup unsweetened orange juice

3 cups all-purpose flour

3 1/2 teaspoons baking powder

1/2 teaspoon salt

Grated rind of one orange

Cooking spray

Preheat oven to 350°. Place sugar, margarine, and egg in large bowl and combine with an electric mixer. Fold in milk and juice. In a separate bowl, sift together flour, baking powder, and salt. Mix dry ingredients into wet ingredients. Stir in orange rind and pour batter into large loaf pan coated with cooking spray. Bake for 47 minutes, or until a toothpick inserted into the center of the loaf comes out clean. Turn out of loaf pan to cool.

Makes 17 (1/2-inch-thick slice) servings
Preparation time: 15 minutes
Baking time: 47 minutes

Nutrient Information (per serving):

Servings per recipe 17

Serving size 1 slice

Carbohydrate choices 2

Calories 129

Carbohydrate 27 grams

Protein 3 grams

Fat 1 gram

Saturated Fat <1 gram

Cholesterol 13 milligrams

Sodium 177 milligrams

Dietary Fiber 1 gram

% calories from:

Protein 9%

Carbohydrate 84%

Fat 7%

Food Exchanges: 1 starch, 1 fruit

Cinnamon Apple-Raisin Cake

Try using Rome Beauty apples in this cake. The Rome Beauty is a red-skinned apple that is particularly good for baking and available nearly year-round.

1/4 cup sugar

1/4 cup + 2 tablespoons packed brown sugar

4 tablespoons reduced-calorie stick margarine

2 egg whites

1/2 cup skim milk

1 1/2 cups all-purpose flour

2 teaspoons baking powder

1/4 teaspoon salt

1 teaspoon cinnamon

1/2 cup seedless golden raisins

1 cup diced apple

Cooking spray

1/2 apple, cored and sliced in thin rings

1/8 teaspoon cinnamon

Preheat oven to 375°. Place sugars, margarine, and egg whites in a large bowl and mix together using an electric mixer. Add milk and mix again. In a separate bowl, sift together flour, baking powder, salt, and 1 teaspoon cinnamon. Stir dry ingredients into wet ingredients. Add raisins and diced apple and stir once again. Place batter in a 9" x 9" baking pan coated with cooking spray. Arrange apple rings on top of batter, press in slightly, and sprinkle with remaining 1/8 teaspoon cinnamon. Bake for 25 to 30 minutes, or until toothpick inserted into center of cake comes out clean. Serve warm.

Makes 9 (1 square) servings
Preparation time: 15 minutes
Baking time: 30 minutes

Nutrient Information (per serving):

Servings per recipe 9
Serving size 1 3-inch square
Carbohydrate choices 3
Calories 207
Carbohydrate 41 grams
Protein 4 grams
Fat 3 grams
Saturated Fat 1 gram

Cholesterol <1 milligram
Sodium 249 milligrams
Dietary Fiber 1 gram
% calories from:
  Protein 8%
  Carbohydrate 79%
  Fat 13%

Food Exchanges: 2 starch, 1 fruit

Creamy Banana Custard

A custard that is so rich-tasting you won't even miss the cream, whole eggs, and sugar of traditional custard! The purpose of scalding the milk in this recipe is to shorten the baking time.

1 cup skim milk

1/2 cup liquid egg substitute

1 teaspoon vanilla

1 drop yellow food coloring

1/2 teaspoon cinnamon

1 1/2 small very ripe bananas, mashed well

1 teaspoon brown sugar

Preheat oven to 300°. Scald milk and cool 10 minutes.

Place egg substitute in a small mixing bowl. Add 2 tablespoons scalded milk to the egg substitute while whisking constantly. Add another 2 tablespoons scalded milk to the egg mixture, again whisking constantly. Pour remaining scalded milk in a large mixing bowl. Add egg mixture, vanilla, food coloring, cinnamon, and mashed bananas to this remaining scalded milk; beat well with electric mixer. Pour mixture into 4 custard cups. Place cups in a pan of hot water that is 1-inch deep. Bake for 50 minutes, or until a knife inserted near the edge of the custard comes out clean. Remove custards from pan of water, sprinkle each with 1/4 teaspoon brown sugar, and allow to cool on a rack.

Note: To scald milk, place milk in a saucepan over medium-high heat and cook, stirring frequently, until tiny bubbles form around the edge of the pan and the milk reaches 180 degrees.

Makes 4 (1/2 cup) servings
Preparation time: 25 minutes
Baking time: 50 minutes

Nutrient Information (per serving):

Servings per recipe 4
Serving size 1/2 cup
Carbohydrate choices 1
Calories 93
Carbohydrate 15 grams
Protein 6 grams
Fat 1 gram
Saturated Fat <1 gram

Cholesterol 1 milligram
Sodium 88 milligrams
Dietary Fiber 1 gram
% calories from:
 Protein 26%
 Carbohydrate 65%
 Fat 10%

Food Exchanges: 1 skim milk

Royal Raisin Rice Pudding

Brown sugar lends a rich caramel color to this version of an old favorite.

3 Choices

1 cup water
1/8 teaspoon salt
2 teaspoons reduced-calorie margarine
1/2 cup medium-grain white rice
1 1/3 cups skim milk
1/3 cup packed brown sugar
1 teaspoon vanilla extract
3/4 cup liquid egg substitute
1/3 cup raisins
1 tablespoon reduced-calorie margarine
Cooking spray
1/4 cup brown sugar
1/2 teaspoon cinnamon

Preheat oven to 325°. Bring water to boil in a large saucepan. Add salt and 2 teaspoons margarine. Stir in rice. Cover and cook over low heat for 15 minutes, or until water is absorbed and rice is tender.

Meanwhile, combine milk, 1/3 cup brown sugar, vanilla extract, egg substitute, and raisins. Add remaining 1 tablespoon margarine to rice and then add egg mixture. Stir well. Pour in baking dish coated with cooking spray. Bake for 45 to 50 minutes, or until pudding is set. Remove from oven and sprinkle with remaining brown sugar and cinnamon.

Makes 6 (1 cup) servings
Preparation time: 20 minutes
Baking time: 50 minutes

Nutrient Information (per serving):

Servings per recipe 6

Serving size 1 cup

Carbohydrate choices 3

Calories 235

Carbohydrate 45 grams

Protein 7 grams

Fat 3 grams

Saturated Fat 1 gram

Cholesterol 1 milligram

Sodium 175 milligrams

Dietary Fiber <1 gram

% calories from:

Protein 12%

Carbohydrate 77%

Fat 11%

Food Exchanges: 2 starch, 1 fruit

Strawberry Banana Spectacular

1½ Choices

*A spectacular light dessert! Top with whole strawberries
for a beautiful finishing touch!*

2 0.3-ounce packages sugar-free strawberry gelatin

2 cups boiling water

2 10-ounce packages sliced frozen strawberries, no sugar added

3 medium bananas, mashed

1 1/2 cups light whipped topping

40 reduced-fat vanilla wafers

In a large bowl, dissolve gelatin in boiling water. Add frozen strawberries to gelatin and stir until berries are thawed. Mix in bananas and place gelatin in refrigerator until slightly thickened, but not set; about 5 minutes. Add whipped topping and stir until combined.

Line a 2-quart serving dish with 20 vanilla wafers and pour half of gelatin mixture over them. Top with remaining 20 vanilla wafers and then remaining gelatin mixture. Cover with plastic wrap and refrigerate 8 hours or overnight.

Makes 15 (1/2 cup) servings
Preparation time: 20 minutes
Chilling time: 8 hours

Nutrient Information (per serving):

Servings per recipe 15

Serving size 1/2 cup

Carbohydrate choices 1 1/2

Calories 102

Carbohydrate 19 grams

Protein 2 grams

Fat 2 grams

Saturated Fat 1 gram

Cholesterol 0

Sodium 50 milligrams

Dietary Fiber 2 grams

% calories from:

Protein 8%

Carbohydrate 75%

Fat 18%

Food Exchanges: 1 starch

Raspberry Trifle with Essence of Mango

2½ Choices

The hint of mango flavor in this delightful trifle comes from mango nectar. Mango nectar is derived from the juice and pulp of the fruit. Small cans of mango nectar can usually be found in the fruit juice section of the grocery store.

- 1 angel food cake, broken into bite-size pieces
- 6 ounces mango nectar
- 10-ounce jar red raspberry 100% fruit spread
- 0.9-ounce package sugar-free vanilla instant pudding, prepared with skim milk
- 3 drops red food coloring
- 8-ounce container light whipped topping
- 1/4 cup finely chopped walnuts

Line a trifle dish with half of the cake pieces. Drizzle cake pieces with half of the mango nectar. Spread with preserves and then pudding. Top with remaining cake pieces and drizzle with remaining nectar. In a separate small bowl, whisk food coloring into whipped topping to tint it pink. Top trifle with pink whipped topping and then sprinkle with walnuts. Refrigerate 8 hours or overnight for best flavor.

Makes 9 (1 cup) servings
Preparation time: 20 minutes
Chilling time: 8 hours

Nutrient Information (per serving):

Servings per recipe 9
Serving size 1 cup
Carbohydrate choices 2 1/2
Calories 209
Carbohydrate 37 grams
Protein 4 grams
Fat 5 grams
Saturated Fat 4 grams

Cholesterol 4 milligrams
Sodium 291 milligrams
Dietary Fiber 4 grams
% calories from:
  Protein 8%
  Carbohydrate 71%
  Fat 22%

Food Exchanges: 1 starch, 1 1/2 fruit, 1 fat

Piña Colada Dessert Creation

Savor the flavors of coconut and pineapple in this light dessert that is reminiscent of the piña colada cocktail.

3 cups fine cinnamon graham cracker crumbs

6 tablespoons reduced-calorie margarine, melted

Cooking spray

2 15 1/4-ounce cans crushed pineapple, packed in juice

3 cups skim milk

1 1/2 teaspoons rum extract

2 1-ounce packages sugar-free instant vanilla pudding mix

3/4 cup flaked coconut, lightly toasted

8-ounce container light whipped topping

4 tablespoons flaked coconut, lightly toasted

In a large bowl, stir together graham cracker crumbs and margarine until crumbs are moistened. Press crumbs into the bottom of a 9" x 13" pan coated with cooking spray. Set aside. In a sieve, drain pineapple well, using a spoon to force out extra juice. Reserve 1/2 cup juice. In a large bowl, combine milk, rum extract, and pudding mix using an electric mixer. Beat on lowest speed for 1 minute. Stir in pineapple, reserved 1/2 cup pineapple juice, and 3/4 cup toasted coconut. Spread filling over crust and refrigerate at least 2 hours.

Before serving, spread whipped topping evenly over filling and sprinkle with remaining 4 tablespoons toasted coconut.

Makes 15 (1 square) servings
Preparation time: 20 minutes
Chilling time: 2 hours

Nutrient Information (per serving):

Servings per recipe 15	Cholesterol 1 milligram
Serving size 1 square	Sodium 242 milligrams
Carbohydrate choices 2 1/2	Dietary Fiber 1 gram
Calories 224	% calories from:
Carbohydrate 34 grams	Protein 7%
Protein 4 grams	Carbohydrate 61%
Fat 8 grams	Fat 32%
Saturated Fat 4 grams	

Food Exchanges: 1 starch, 1 fruit, 1 fat

Berry Good Cheesecake

A simple no-bake cheesecake made in a 9" x 13" pan rather than a springform pan.

Crust:

2 cups graham cracker crumbs

2 packets saccharin sweetener

4 tablespoons reduced-calorie stick margarine, melted

Cooking spray

Filling:

1/4-ounce envelope unflavored gelatin

1 cup skim milk

2 8-ounce packages reduced-fat cream cheese, softened

1/3 cup honey

1/3 cup unsweetened frozen orange juice concentrate

1 teaspoon lemon juice

1/2 teaspoon orange extract

1/2 teaspoon vanilla extract

Topping:

1/4 cup blueberry 100% fruit spread

1/4 cup orange marmalade 100% fruit spread

2 cups fresh blueberries

In a large bowl, combine graham cracker crumbs, sweetener, and margarine. Press crumb mixture into the bottom of a 9" x 13" pan coated with cooking spray. Set aside.

In a small saucepan, whisk together gelatin and milk and let stand 3 minutes. Place over low-medium heat and whisk constantly until gelatin is dissolved and steam rises from milk, but milk does not boil. Remove from heat and cool 5 minutes.

In a large mixing bowl, beat cream cheese with an electric mixer until fluffy. Gradually beat in gelatin mixture, then honey, orange juice concentrate, lemon juice, and extracts. Place in refrigerator and chill about 30 minutes, or until thickened. Spoon mixture over crust and return to refrigerator for 2 1/2 hours, or until filling is set.

To prepare topping, mix together fruit spreads in a medium bowl. Gently stir in blueberries and refrigerate until serving time. Serve a spoonful of topping over each piece of cheesecake.

Makes 15 servings
Preparation time: 30 minutes
Chilling time: 3 hours

Nutrient Information (per serving):

Servings per recipe 15

Serving size 1 square

Carbohydrate choices 1 1/2

Calories 171

Carbohydrate 22 grams

Protein 5 grams

Fat 7 grams

Saturated Fat 4 grams

Cholesterol 11 milligrams

Sodium 237 milligrams

Dietary Fiber <1 gram

% calories from:

Protein 12%

Carbohydrate 51%

Fat 37%

Food Exchanges: 1 whole milk, 1/2 fruit

Red, White, and Blue Berry Bake

Let's hear it for the red, white, and blue—raspberries, vanilla yogurt, and blueberries,!

  4 cups fresh raspberries

  4 cups fresh blueberries

  2 cups sugar-free, low-fat vanilla yogurt

  2 teaspoons brown sugar substitute

  Ground cinnamon

Preheat oven on "broil" setting. Place 1/2 cup raspberries and 1/2 cup blueberries in each of 8 oven-proof bowls. Top each with 1/2 cup yogurt, then sprinkle each with 1/4 teaspoon brown sugar substitute and a dash of cinnamon.

Place bowls in oven and broil 3 inches from heat source for 4 minutes. Leave oven cracked during cooking. Serve immediately.

Makes 8 (1 bowl) servings
Preparation time: 5 minutes
Broiling time: 4 minutes

Nutrient Information (per serving):

Servings per recipe 8	Cholesterol 0
Serving size 1 bowl	Sodium 37 milligrams
Carbohydrate choices 2	Dietary Fiber 6 grams
Calories 121	% calories from:
Carbohydrate 25 grams	Protein 10%
Protein 3 grams	Carbohydrate 83%
Fat <1 gram	Fat 7%
Saturated Fat <1 gram	

Food Exchanges: 2 fruit

Spiced Broiled Peaches

Eat these flavorful peaches alone, or sliced and served warm over sugar-free vanilla ice cream or sugar-free vanilla frozen yogurt.

8 canned peach halves packed in juice, drained
Cooking spray
4 teaspoons reduced-calorie margarine
2 teaspoons brown sugar substitute
1 teaspoon cinnamon
1/2 teaspoon ground nutmeg

Preheat broiler. Place peaches halves in a baking dish coated with cooking spray, sliced side up. Put 1/2 teaspoon margarine in the center of each peach half, then sprinkle with brown sugar substitute, cinnamon, and nutmeg. Place 5 inches from heat source and broil for 5 minutes, or until margarine is melted.

Makes 8 (1/2 peach) servings
Preparation time: 5 minutes
Broiling time: 5 minutes

Nutrient Information (per serving):

Servings per recipe 8

Serving size 1/2 peach

Carbohydrate choices 1

Calories 53

Carbohydrate 10 grams

Protein 1 gram

Fat 1 gram

Saturated Fat <1 gram

Cholesterol 0

Sodium 26 milligrams

Dietary Fiber 1 gram

% calories from:

   Protein 8%

   Carbohydrate 75%

   Fat 17%

Food Exchanges: 1 fruit

Apple Cider Sauce

This unique sauce is a great topper, hot or cold, for sugar-free vanilla ice cream or gingerbread. Store the leftovers in the refrigerator to use later for a quick special treat!

1 tablespoon + 2 teaspoons reduced-calorie margarine

1 tablespoon + 1 teaspoon all-purpose flour

2 1/4 cups apple cider

1 1/2 teaspoons ground cinnamon

1/4 teaspoon ground cloves

Melt margarine in saucepan over medium heat. Mix in flour with a wire whisk and simmer until thickened. Whisk in cider and spices. Increase heat and bring to a boil. Boil for 1 minute, or until sauce is the consistency of honey.

Makes 8 (1/4 cup) servings
Preparation time: 5 minutes

Nutrient Information (per serving):

Servings per recipe 8

Serving size 1/4 cup

Carbohydrate choices 1

Calories 57

Carbohydrate 11 grams

Protein <1 gram

Fat 1 gram

Saturated Fat <1 gram

Cholesterol 0

Sodium 31 milligrams

Dietary Fiber <1 gram

% calories from:

Protein 7%

Carbohydrate 77%

Fat 16%

Food Exchanges: 1 fruit

Raspberry-Orange Sauce

Delightful served over sugar-free vanilla ice cream, angel food cake, or a slice of fresh cantaloupe.

1
Choice

10-ounce jar red raspberry 100% fruit spread
1 tablespoon fresh grated orange rind
1/3 cup unsweetened orange juice
1 1/2 tablespoons orange liqueur
1 cup fresh raspberries

In a large bowl, combine raspberry spread, orange rind, orange juice, and orange liqueur. Gently stir in raspberries. May chill before serving if desired.

Makes 8 (1/4 cup) servings
Preparation time: 5 minutes

Nutrient Information (per serving):

Servings per recipe 8
Serving size 1/4 cup
Carbohydrate choices 1
Calories 69
Carbohydrate 14 grams
Protein <1 gram
Fat <1 gram
Saturated Fat 0

Cholesterol 0
Sodium 42 milligrams
Dietary Fiber 1 gram
% calories from:
  Protein 6%
  Carbohydrate 81%
  Fat 13%

Food Exchanges: 1 fruit

Sample Menus

For an 1800-calorie Meal Plan

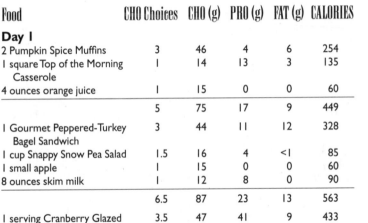

Food	CHO Choices	CHO (g)	PRO (g)	FAT (g)	CALORIES
Day 1					
2 Pumpkin Spice Muffins	3	46	4	6	254
1 square Top of the Morning Casserole	1	14	13	3	135
4 ounces orange juice	1	15	0	0	60
	5	75	17	9	449
1 Gourmet Peppered-Turkey Bagel Sandwich	3	44	11	12	328
1 cup Snappy Snow Pea Salad	1.5	16	4	<1	85
1 small apple	1	15	0	0	60
8 ounces skim milk	1	12	8	0	90
	6.5	87	23	13	563
1 serving Cranberry Glazed Sirloin Tips over Noodles	3.5	47	41	9	433
1/2 cup Brown Sugar Butternut Squash	1.5	16	2	7	135
1 Cream-Filled Chocolate Cupcake	1.5	19	2	4	120
8 ounces skim milk	1	12	8	0	90
	7.5	94	53	20	778
TOTAL	19	256	93	42	1790

Food	CHO Choices	CHO (g)	PRO (g)	FAT (g)	CALORIES
Day 2					
Cinnamon Spice Instant Oatmeal (1 packet)	2.5	35	5	2	177
1 teaspoon margarine	0	0	0	5	45
2 Cheesy Ham and Mushroom Quiche Bites	1	10	12	4	124
1 cup strawberries	1	15	0	0	60
8 ounces low-fat milk	1	12	8	5	120
	5.5	72	25	16	526
1 cup Spaghetti Salad Supreme	2.5	33	6	3	183
1 serving Garlic Parmesan Pull-Apart Bread	2	29	5	5	181
1.5 cups fresh fruit salad	1.5	23	0	0	90
8 ounces Lemon Mint Tea-ser	0	1	<1	<1	4
	6	86	12	9	458
1 Chicken & Mushroom Bundle	2	27	15	18	330
1 cup Quick Broccoli Parmesano	1	9	5	3	83
1/2 cup Country Corn Pudding	2	24	9	4	168
1 Easy Refrigerator Bar	1.5	16	3	3	103
8 ounces low-fat milk	1	12	8	5	120
	7.5	88	40	33	804
TOTAL	19	246	77	58	1788
Day 3					
2 Berry Patch Muffins	3	38	6	6	230
1.5 cups fresh cantaloupe	1.5	23	0	0	90
8 ounces skim milk	1	12	8	0	90
	5.5	73	14	6	410
2 slices Western-Style Chicken Pizza	4.5	67	36	13	529
2 chocolate chip cookies	1	15	1	4	100
Diet soft drink	0	0	0	0	0
	5.5	82	37	17	629
4 ounces Aloha Orange Roughy	0	4	22	3	131
1 cup Seasoned Wild Rice with Mushrooms	3	44	6	4	236
1 serving Basil and Chive Tomato Bake	1	14	9	11	191
1 square Berry Good Cheesecake	1.5	22	5	7	171
8 ounces skim milk	1	12	8	0	90
	6.5	96	50	25	819
TOTAL	18.5	251	101	48	1858

Recipe Listings

~

Recipes Grouped by Number of Carbohydrate Choices per Serving

0 Choices

Beverages
Cranberry Sparkler
Icy Cinnamon Cafe
Lemon Mint Tea-ser

Appetizers
Asparagus in Tangy Dijon Vinaigrette
Buffalo Chicken Bites
Cocktail Chicken Spread
Favorite Chipped Beef Spread

Great Gazpacho Dip
Italian Artichoke Dip
New England Crab Spread
Rich Broccoli and Cheese Dip

Salads
Colorful Ranch-Style Salad
Creamy Orange Gelatin
Overnight Marinated Vegetable Salad

Entrées
Aloha Orange Roughy
Diablo Shrimp
Dijon-Basted Pork Tenderloin
Herb Roasted Chicken
Peppery Beef Roast with Gravy

1/2 Choice

Beverages
Tomato Basil Warm-Up

Appetizers
Cheesy Ham and Mushroom Quiche Bites
South-of-the-Border Dip
Tasty Tortilla Roll-Ups

Salads
Chinese Sprout Salad
Crispy Cucumbers and Onions

Herbed Tomato Slices
Oriental Chicken Salad
Strawberry Spinach Salad with Toasted Almonds

Entrées
Marjoram Baked Halibut with Parmesan Crumb Topping
Sensational Stuffed Flounder

Side Dishes
Creole Cabbage
Dilled Peas, Carrots, and Pearl Onions
Dilly-Lemon Glazed Baby Carrots
Green Bean Saute
Grilled Eggplant Oregano

Desserts
No-Bake Peanut Butter Cookies

1 Choice

Beverages
Frosty Orange Frappe

Appetizers
Chilled Cucumber Soup
Quick Hummus Dip

Salads
Cinnamon Apple-Raisin Slaw
Greco-Italian Tossed Salad
Picante Red-Skin Potato Salad

Entrées
Layered Chicken Salad Ole

Mediterranean Eggplant Bake
Pizza Meat Loaf
Stuffed Cabbage Leaves with Tomato Sauce
Tender Pork Chops with Mushroom Gravy
Teriyaki Pork Kabobs
Texas Tortilla Soup
Top of the Morning Casserole
Turkey Cutlets in White Wine Sauce

Side Dishes
Basil and Chive Tomato Bake

Pineapple Glazed Beets
Quick Broccoli Parmesano
Savory Black Bean and Shoepeg Corn Salsa
Summer Squash Saute
Tangy Cauliflower Toss

Desserts
Apple Cider Sauce
Banana-Pineapple Confection
Creamy Banana Custard
Raspberry Orange Sauce
Spiced Broiled Peaches
Thumbprint Cookies

1 1/2 Choices

Appetizers
Mini Pita Pizzas
Spicy Tortilla Chips

Breads
Berry Patch Muffins
Broccoli Cheese Bread
Pumpkin Spice Muffins
Ready-in-a-Flash Rolls

Salads
Snappy Snow Pea Salad
Spicy Southwestern Bean Salad

Entrées
Barbecue Vegetable Pita Pockets
Easy Vegetable Quiche
Sauteed Sea Scallops with Angel Hair Pasta
Spinach and Ham Bow Tie Pasta

Side Dishes
Brown Sugar Butternut Squash
Corny Tomato Boats
Great Northern Beans with Garlic and Rosemary
Mom's Old-Fashioned Baked Beans

Rosemary Red-Skin Potatoes and Sugar Snap Peas
Spicy Three-Bean Combo
Tangy Marinated Carrot Coins

Desserts
Berry Good Cheesecake
Cream-Filled Chocolate Cupcakes
Easy Refrigerator Bars
Strawberry Banana Spectacular
Summer Strawberry Mousse

2 Choices

Breads
Garlic Parmesan Pull-Apart Bread

Entrées
Cantina Pasta Salad
Chicken & Mushroom Bundles
Chicken and Broccoli Deluxe

Confetti Tamale Casserole
Fiesta Chicken Picante
Navy Bean and Ham Soup
Tuna and Shells Toss

Side Dishes
Angel Hair Pasta, Mediterranean-Style
Cherry Walnut Brown Rice

Country Corn Pudding
Crispy Oven "Fries"

Desserts
Orange Delight Dessert Loaf
Red, White, and Blue Berry Bake

2 1/2 Choices

Salads
Pineapple Jubilee
Spaghetti Salad Supreme

Entrées
Sicilian Spinach-Potato Bake
Turkey for Two in Foil

Turkey Parmesan
Under the Sea Sandwich

Side Dishes
Garlic and Chive Mashed Potatoes

Desserts
Kahlua Ice Cream Dessert
Pina Colada Dessert Creation
Raspberry Trifle with Essence of Mango
Triple Chocolate Parfait

3 Choices

Entrées
Chargrilled Steak and Potatoes on a Stick
Chili Italiano
Gourmet Peppered-Turkey Bagel Sandwich

Side Dishes
Greek Broiled Potatoes
Seasoned Wild Rice with Mushrooms
Sensational Stuffed Sweet Potatoes

Desserts
Cinnamon Apple-Raisin Cake
Royal Raisin Rice Pudding

3 1/2 Choices

Entrées
Cranberry Glazed Sirloin Tips over Noodles
Polish Sausage Skillet Supper

4 Choices

Entrées
Chinese Pepper Pork
Spicy Black Bean and Rice Soup
Veggie Jambalaya

4 1/2 Choices

Entrées
Western-Style Chicken Pizza

Recipes Grouped by Number of Grams of Carbohydrate per Serving

0–15 Grams

Beverages
Cranberry Sparkler 4g
Frosty Orange Frappe 10g
Icy Cinnamon Cafe 2g
Lemon Mint Tea-ser 1g
Tomato Basil Warm-Up 8g

Appetizers
Asparagus in Tangy Dijon Vinaigrette 3g
Buffalo Chicken Bites 1g
Cheesy Ham and Mushroom Quiche Bites 5g
Chilled Cucumber Soup 13g
Cocktail Chicken Spread 1g
Favorite Chipped Beef Spread 1g
Great Gazpacho Dip 2g
Italian Artichoke Dip 4g
New England Crab Spread 1g
Quick Hummus Dip 12g
Rich Broccoli and Cheese Dip 2g
South-of-the-Border Dip 7g
Tasty Tortilla Roll-Ups 8g

Salads
Chinese Sprout Salad 7g
Cinnamon Apple-Raisin Slaw 9g
Colorful Ranch-Style Salad 4g
Creamy Orange Gelatin 3g
Crispy Cucumbers and Onions 6g
Greco-Italian Tossed Salad 12g
Herbed Tomato Slices 5g
Oriental Chicken Salad 6g
Overnight Marinated Vegetable Salad 4g
Picante Red-Skin Potato Salad 10g
Strawberry Spinach Salad with Toasted Almonds 5g

Entrées
Aloha Orange Roughy 4g
Diablo Shrimp 1g
Dijon-Basted Pork Tenderloin 1g
Herb-Roasted Chicken 1g
Layered Chicken Salad Ole 12g
Marjoram Baked Halibut with Parmesan Crumb Topping 6g
Mediterranean Eggplant Bake 10g
Peppery Beef Roast with Gravy 3g
Pizza Meat Loaf 9g
Sensational Stuffed Flounder 8g
Stuffed Cabbage Leaves with Tomato Sauce 12g
Tender Pork Chops with Mushroom Gravy 10g
Teriyaki Pork Kabobs 13g
Texas Tortilla Soup 12g
Top of the Morning Casserole 14g
Turkey Cutlets in White Wine Sauce 11g

Side Dishes
Basil and Chive Tomato Bake 14g
Creole Cabbage 7g
Dilled Peas, Carrots, and Pearl Onions 8g
Dilly-Lemon Glazed Baby Carrots 6g
Green Bean Sauté 5g
Grilled Eggplant Oregano 6g
Pineapple Glazed Beets 14g
Quick Broccoli Parmesano 9g
Savory Black Bean and Shoepeg Corn Salsa 11g
Summer Squash Sauté 9g
Tangy Cauliflower Toss 9g

Desserts
Apple Cider Sauce 11g
Banana-Pineapple Confection 15g
Creamy Banana Custard 15g
No-Bake Peanut Butter Cookies 7g
Raspberry-Orange Sauce 14g
Spiced Broiled Peaches 10g
Thumbprint Cookies 10g

16–30 Grams

Appetizers
Mini Pita Pizzas 22g
Spicy Tortilla Chips 17g

Breads
Berry Patch Muffins 19g
Broccoli Cheese Bread 16g
Garlic Parmesan Pull-Apart Bread 29g
Pumpkin Spice Muffins 23g
Ready-in-a-Flash Rolls 17g

Salads
Snappy Snow Pea Salad 16g
Spicy Southwestern Bean Salad 22g

Entrées
Barbecue Vegetable Pita Pockets 22g
Cantina Pasta Salad 25g
Chicken & Mushroom Bundles 27g
Chicken and Broccoli Deluxe 26g
Confetti Tamale Casserole 29g
Easy Vegetable Quiche 16g
Fiesta Chicken Picante 28g
Navy Bean and Ham Soup 30g
Sautéed Sea Scallops with Angel Hair Pasta 23g
Spinach and Ham Bow Tie Pasta 19g
Tuna and Shells Toss 25g

Side Dishes
Angel Hair Pasta, Mediterranean Style 27g
Brown Sugar Butternut Squash 16g
Cherry Walnut Brown Rice 29g
Corny Tomato Boats 22g
Country Corn Pudding 24g
Crispy Oven "Fries" 29g
Great Northern Beans with Garlic and Rosemary 23g
Mom's Old-Fashioned Baked Beans 23g
Rosemary Red-Skin Potatoes and Sugar Snap Peas 22g
Spicy Three-Bean Combo 20g
Tangy Marinated Carrot Coins 20g

Desserts
Berry Good Cheesecake 22g
Cream-Filled Chocolate Cupcakes 19g
Easy Refrigerator Bars 16g
Orange Delight Dessert Loaf 27g
Red, White and Blue Berry Bake 25g
Strawberry Banana Spectacular 19g
Summer Strawberry Mousse 18g

31–45 Grams

Salads
Pineapple Jubilee 33g
Spaghetti Salad Supreme 33g

Entrées
Chargrilled Steak and Potatoes on a Stick 43g
Chili Italiano 45g
Gourmet Peppered-Turkey Bagel Sandwich 44g
Sicilian Spinach-Potato Bake 38g
Turkey for Two in Foil 34g
Turkey Parmesan 31g
Under the Sea Sandwich 34g

Side Dishes
Garlic and Chive Mashed Potatoes 35g
Greek Broiled Potatoes 39g
Seasoned Wild Rice with Mushrooms 44g
Sensational Stuffed Sweet Potatoes 41g

Desserts
Cinnamon Apple-Raisin Cake 41g
Kahlua Ice Cream Dessert 35g
Pina Colada Dessert Creation 34g
Raspberry Trifle with Essence of Mango 37g
Royal Raisin Rice Pudding 45g
Triple Chocolate Parfait 38g

46–60 Grams

Entrées:
Chinese Pepper Pork: 55g
Cranberry Glazed Sirloin Tips over Noodles: 47g
Polish Sausage Skillet Supper: 53g
Spicy Black Bean and Rice Soup: 59g
Veggie Jambalaya: 55g

Over 61 Grams

Entrées:
Western-Style Chicken Pizza: 67g

Index

Also from John Wiley & Sons

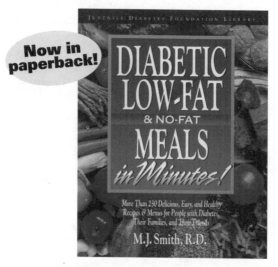

Also from John Wiley & Sons

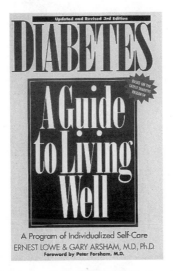

Diabetes: A Guide to Living Well
Third Edition
Ernest Lowe and Gary Arsham, MD, PhD

The third edition of *Diabetes: A Guide to Living Well* incorporates new information learned about diabetes since the last edition, emphasizing the current focus on preventive measures to avoid complications. For the first time, the book also includes helpful advice for managing Type 2 diabetes.

Available at your favorite bookstore.